Breast Cancer

Taking Control

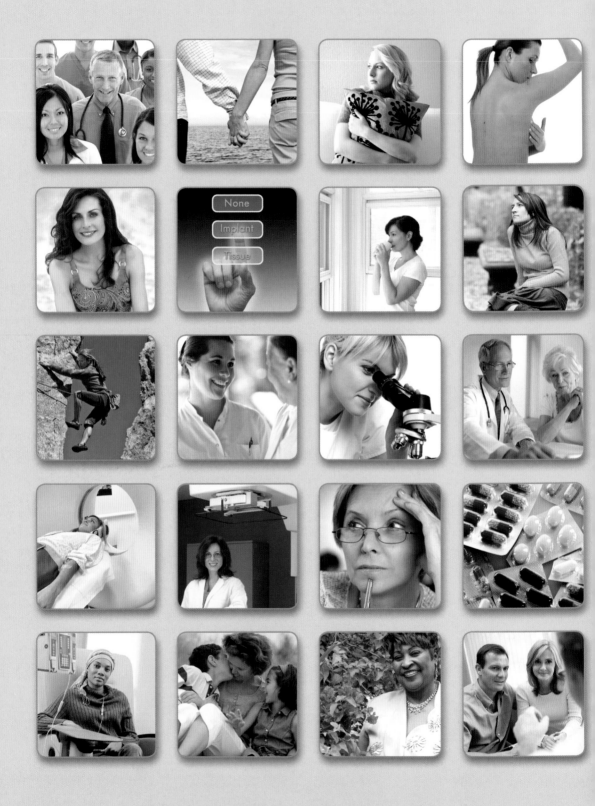

Breast Cancer

Taking Control

Professor John Boyages, MD, PhD

Boycare Publishing

Sydney, Australia

Praise for Breast Cancer: Taking Control

"The results from the biopsy are back, and I'm afraid you have breast cancer." How many countless of thousands of women have heard these words and felt the bottom drop out of their lives? For many, these words are taken as a death sentence—and certainly for all they mean the beginning of an often painful series of treatments and a long and arduous journey to recovery.

Arguably, breast cancer has touched more patients and their families than any other malignancy due to its common incidence, its occurrence in so many younger women with families and loved ones who depend on them, and the necessity of treatments that affect fundamental issues of femininity, sexuality, and cosmetics. Yet, there is good news. Over the last 30 years, statistics from most developed countries have demonstrated that in spite of the increasing incidence of the disease, overall mortality has dropped dramatically, due to screening, early detection, and better treatments, especially if applied, immediately after surgery, in the 'adjuvant' setting.

Furthermore, medical advances have led to less-disfiguring surgery and less-toxic radiation and systemic therapies. Unfortunately, these exciting results require that a patient and her family work through a complicated maze of treatment options and strategies. They also raise important issues regarding how to deal with entirely new and, for most women, unfamiliar strategies to get the best treatment possible while minimizing side effects and long-term toxicities.

Which is where *Breast Cancer: Taking Control* comes in. Dr. John Boyages brings to bear his considerable experiences and skills, obtained during training and a clinical practice devoted to the care and study of breast cancer. His efforts span nearly three decades and two continents. There are many books on the lay market for a patient with breast cancer. However, few are written with such a folksy and sympathetic approach as this one.

I have had the wonderful opportunity to observe Dr. Boyages's career unfold, and I am not surprised by the quality of this resource. He has always been a great doctor, taking a "what if you were my family member" approach, and this spirit shines throughout this book. Perhaps the greatest compliment one doctor can have for another is that "He (or she) is the one I'd have take care of me."

I'd be pleased to have John take care of any member of my own family, and if they had breast cancer, I'd certainly recommend that they read this book—-and so I recommend it to you as well!

—**Daniel F. Hayes, MD**

Stuart A. Padnos Professor of Breast Cancer Research
University of Michigan Comprehensive Cancer Center
Ann Arbor

I want to thank you very much for sending me your e-book just after I was diagnosed with early breast cancer. I read it cover to cover (so to speak) in two sittings the weekend you sent it. I must tell you: it was tremendously helpful to me. I particularly liked the fact that you explained the statistics in an intuitive and easy-to-grasp way, and that you gave all the relevant figures. Speaking as a philosopher of psychology, it was good that you mostly put things in terms of frequencies— this is the way that human beings can best think about this sort of information. Well done!

—Fiona Cowie

Associate Professor of Philosophy
California Institute of Technology

Dr. John Boyages is an innovator amongst his peers; he is unafraid to address the unique and sensitive issues that many breast cancer survivors are facing on a day to day basis. Concerns about quality of life, fertility preservation, sexual health and wellness, and menopause are often neglected in the comprehensive care of the cancer patient. Yet Dr. Boyages addresses these concerns with compassion and medical accuracy. The book provides clear, understandable solutions that put the reader at ease. It is an excellent resource for patients and caregivers and a first-rate addition to the oncology, sexual medicine, and cancer survivorship fields.

—**Michael L. Krychman, MD**

Medical Director of Sexual Medicine Hoag Hospital,
Executive Director of the Southern California Center for Sexual Health
and Survivorship Medicine,
Associate Clinical Professor University of Southern California

John Boyages is one of those few oncologists who understands all aspects of breast cancer. He is a doctor's doctor who treats many doctors and their families. This is a must-read, not only for women with breast cancer but also for oncology trainees, nurses, and general practitioners.

— **Richard Kefford, MD**

Professor of Medicine, Medical Oncologist and Director of the Westmead Institute for Cancer
Research University of Sydney Department of Medicine,
Westmead Hospital

John Boyages is absolutely right: women do remember the first three months after initial diagnosis of breast cancer as the most confusing and frightening. I did. This is the first book to acknowledge and address that, and it is most welcome. This comprehensive yet personal guide will help women to feel that they can handle their [treatment] decisions because it gives them the information they need at the right time, and in one place.

—**Sally Crossing, AM**

Founding Chair, Breast Cancer Action Group NSW

An easy read for a layperson without a medical background—insightful and informative.

—**Michelle Hanton OAM**

Founder Dragons Abreast Australia

Nobody wants to hear the words "You have cancer." But Professor John Boyages has helped many women not just survive but thrive after the heartbreak of a breast cancer diagnosis. John is a leader in multidisciplinary care and sees patients from all over the world. Apart from his clinical work, he is also a passionate advocate for breast cancer education, and whenever journalists need help with a breast cancer story, he responds promptly and always in plain English, without medical gobbledygook! John has won several awards for services to medicine and the media, and the tips in this book are a must-read for anyone on the breast cancer journey.

—**Jane Worthington**

Health reporter
Woman's Day, Reader's Digest HealthSmart and The Sunday Telegraph

It has been a great privilege to read through this book, and John Boyages is to be congratulated on the quality and scope of the manuscript. I particularly liked the use of the first person—the tone was just right and it really felt as though he were talking the reader through their diagnosis, treatment, and beyond. This will be an invaluable resource to women with breast cancer and I imagine that they will refer back to it many times during their course of treatment.

— **Elizabeth Salisbury MD**

Senior Staff Specialist and Associate Professor, Department of Anatomical Pathology,
Prince of Wales Hospital, NSW, Australia

I found your book very easy to read. In fact, I read it in a day. It was just as if you were talking with me in person. I really felt the book expressed your genuineness and concern in wanting to help women with breast cancer. The book also helped me to understand what had happened in my life when I was told I had breast cancer. I wish I'd had a copy when I was first diagnosed.

—**Laraine Dick**

About the Author

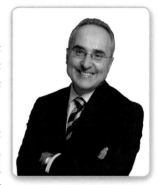

John Boyages, MB BS (Hons), FRACR PhD is a cancer specialist with over 25 years' experience in the diagnosis and treatment of breast cancer. He is a busy clinician who cares for patients at Westmead, the Hills, and the Sydney Adventist hospitals.

Following his training at the University of Sydney and a fellowship at Harvard Medical School under the direction of Professor Jay Harris, he was appointed as a specialist radiation oncologist at Westmead Hospital in 1989 and founded one of the largest free breast cancer screening programs in the west of Sydney.

In 1995, he won a grant to establish and direct the Westmead Breast Cancer Institute, which offers clinical care, research, education, and screening programs. The Institute is a research unit within the Faculty of Medicine at the University of Sydney, where John holds an academic Professorship.

He has published more than 130 research and clinical articles and is committed to the dissemination of research findings to lay and professional audiences both nationally and internationally. To that end, John has worked in partnership with the Breast Cancer Action Group NSW, a patient advocacy group.

John performs numerous national roles in his field, and his current international roles include: member of the International Union Against Cancer (UICC), member of the International Expert Advisory Panel for the Staging of Breast Cancer, invited research collaborator with the United StatesNational Cancer Institute (NCI) on hormone replacement therapy and breast cancer, and member of the editorial board of the *European Journal of Cancer*.

In 2006, John received a national Medical Media Award for outstanding service to the media and the community.

Breast Cancer: Taking Control
Boycare Publishing, Australia
PO Box 568, Beecroft, NSW 2119, Australia
Boycare@gmail.com

National Library of Australia Cataloguing-in-Publication entry: Book

Author: Boyages, John.
Title: Breast cancer : taking control / John Boyages.
Edition: 1st ed.
ISBN: 978-0-9806311-1-1
Subjects: Breast--Cancer.
Breast--Cancer--Patients.
Breast--Cancer--Treatment.
Dewey Number: 616.99449

Library in Congress Control Number: 2010907247

To Dianne, Fiona, and Peter
with love. Thank you for all your
love and support

To the brave women
with breast cancer

Acknowledgments

Firstly, thanks to all my friends, patients, neighbors, colleagues, and others who have helped by spurring me on to produce this work or giving me a lot of their precious time.

I would especially like to thank my wife, Dianne, for her ongoing patience and support and her understanding of the number of hours I spend away from our family pursuing my passion of helping women (and a few men) fight breast cancer. Thanks also to my beautiful children, Fiona and Peter, for their ongoing humor, support, and understanding. Special thanks to my daughter, Fiona Collison, who currently works in the publishing industry, for her critical (and honest) review of the book at key stages of its development.

Thank you to my "patient support team": Margaret Mapperson for her expert help with some of the graphics in this book and her encouragement and Elaine (another breast cancer survivor) and Tony Eccleston for their very helpful suggestions and ongoing support. Special thanks also to Leigh Hatcher and his wife, Meredith, for their critical review of the document, and for spurring me on to complete and simplify the book.

Expert medical review of sections of the book were undertaken by my colleagues Mrs. Elisabeth Black, Mrs. Jenny Cooper, Professor Martha Hickey, Dr. Amanda Hordern, Mrs. Louise Koelmeyer, Dr. Michael Krychman, Dr. Thomas Lam, Dr. James French, Dr. Rina Hui, Dr. Tim Wang, and Associate Professor Nicholas Wilcken. Special thanks to Dr. Steve Kelly and Associate Professor Elizabeth Salisbury for their critical and expert review of the entire book. Thanks to Judy Simon, President and CEO of Nearly Me Technologies, Inc., for her critical review of Control Point #5 regarding prostheses after a mastectomy.

Thanks, too, to my previous teachers at Westmead Hospital and Harvard University for their ability to teach me how to question and learn about this dreaded disease, which is far too common. Thanks also to all my patients who have taught me more than you can believe over the last 25 years in the field of oncology.

Thanks also to Rachel Haimowitz, my US editor, for her expert editing of this work and to Olivia Wroth for proofreading the graphically designed document. Special thanks to Mishu Rahman for putting his heart and soul into the graphic design of this book to ensure that it stands out from the crowd, and more importantly, that women with breast cancer can read it easily during a time of great stress.

Finally, thanks to my late father, Constantine, and mother, Fotini, who migrated from Greece after World War II and taught me the value of hard work, honesty, education, and lifelong learning.

Foreword

The diagnosis of breast cancer is devastating. Following a diagnosis, many people today turn to the Internet to get answers before they see their doctor, but resources on the web are scattered and often inaccurate or unhelpful. At long last, a breast cancer expert has written a book that focuses on what a patient needs to know from the point of diagnosis.

Breast Cancer: Taking Control takes you through all the critical decision points after a diagnosis in a personal, plain English style, and in one place gives you all the information you need.

John Boyages completed a fellowship with me at the Dana-Farber Cancer Institute in 1988, and since then, I have been proud to watch him become one of the world's all-around experts about this complex disease. In this book, John takes you through the treatment journey with empathy, care, and common sense and gives hope and power back to the reader to let them regain control when life seems suddenly so out of control.

Jay R. Harris, MD
Professor, Department of Radiation Oncology, Harvard Medical School
Chief, Radiation Oncology Department, Dana-Farber Cancer Institute

Contents

PART 2: "GAINING CONTROL"
TAKING CONTROL BEFORE YOUR SURGERY

PART 3: "MAINTAINING CONTROL"
TAKING CONTROL AFTER YOUR SURGERY

Patient Stories

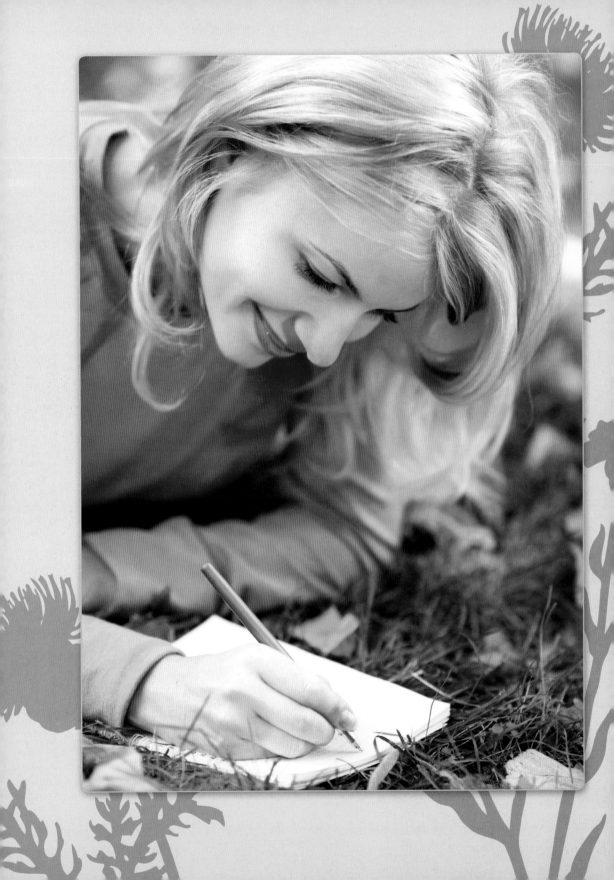

Mel's Story

I didn't sleep for days after my diagnosis. I wasn't expecting to be told I had breast cancer. I found some thickening in my breast and was sent to a radiologist for a mammogram.

The mammogram was normal, and my doctor advised me to "keep an eye on it" for the moment and come back if it changed. I was only 31 at the time.

I went back to the doctor three months later, and again was told not to worry about it. Six months later, I went to a 24-hour medical center and asked for another test. This time, the doctor on duty organized an ultrasound, which showed a very abnormal lump, and a biopsy was done at the same time.

The radiologist told me that he thought it was cancer. I felt helpless and alone. I was in shock and could hardly find my way back to the car. I went back to the medical center and was referred to a surgeon.

It took ten days to get an appointment, and I really thought my life was over. That was ten years ago and life has just got better and better for me every year.

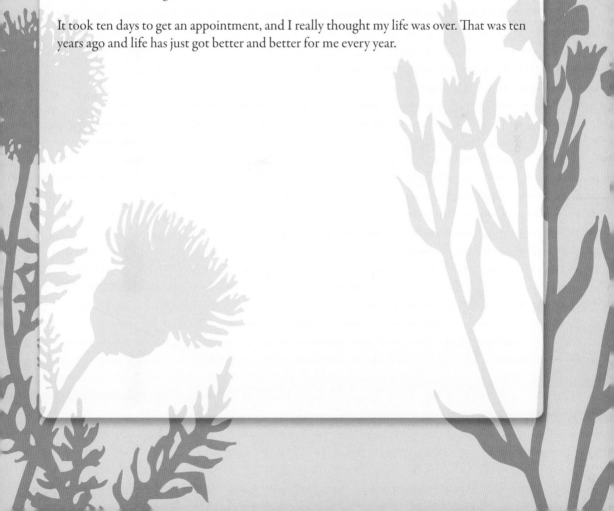

Introduction

Introduction

Hi, my name is Professor John Boyages. Most of my patients call me John. Every week, I see at least ten new patients with breast cancer, and every year I do post-treatment checkups on thousands of others. I have treated many women (and men) with breast cancer, and let me tell you, the first week is the worst. And the first day is usually the worst of all (see "Mel's Story").

In 1983, I decided that helping people with cancer would become an important part of my career. I had some terrible experiences in the early years—doctors, often surgeons, would starkly and insensitively tell their patients they had a "tumor," and "we will refer you to treatment." I was then left to tell them, as gently as I could, what was really going on.

I remember a woman who was dying of pancreatic cancer, and the lead physician would not allow us to tell her so because it would "make it worse." I can't recall what finally made me choose to devote my career to treating patients with cancer, but I have never regretted the decision.

My interest in breast cancer started back in 1983 when my mentor, Professor Alan Langlands, asked me to do some breast cancer research with him during my training. I never looked back.

After graduating from Sydney University with a degree in medicine and another in radiation oncology, I enrolled in a PhD and was invited to do further study at Harvard University. Since then, I have set up various programs in the west of Sydney, including one of the largest breast screening programs internationally. At Harvard, I worked with some of the best masters in the world. I am eternally grateful to leading

MDs Jay Harris, Craig Henderson, Susan Love, Jim Connolly, Stuart Schnitt, Abe Recht, Dan Hayes and many others for allowing me to work with them at the Breast Evaluation Clinic (the "BEC") at the Dana-Farber Cancer Institute and the Beth Israel Deaconess Medical Center in Boston, and for helping me to learn good research practices and recognize good science.

The aim of this book is to help you or your family member

1. Understand what may happen after a diagnosis of breast cancer.

2. Understand not only what treatments are available, but also how best to use them in your own situation.

3. Understand the evidence supporting the treatment choices you may face after a diagnosis, including:

    • Do I really need a **mastectomy**?

    • Is **breast conservation** (removal of your cancerous lump, also known as a **lumpectomy**) the best approach for me?

    • What's the best test for seeing if the cancer has spread to my lymph glands (also known as nodes) under my armpit?

    • Can I get away with not having **chemotherapy**?

    • What are the side effects of all these treatments?

4. Regain control by teaching you the evidence for treatment decisions and dispelling many of the myths.

This book will detail some of my insight and experience into what it's like to treat a patient who has just been diagnosed with breast cancer. It will help you get through the physical and mental strain of the first year or so after your diagnosis. Those first three months are critical for your long-term **prognosis**, because the choices you make during that time can affect the risk of your cancer coming back. Research has shown that being involved in informed choices is important for your sense of wellbeing and control (Morris 1987).

There are many books and websites out there that will tell you what to do. I'll detail some of the best websites (and particularly web links to specific information) throughout this book.

I'm not going to repeat everything; I'll just give you the most important bits in a logical order. The trouble with websites and "support guides" is that they don't know what not to tell you. Basically, they give you too much information, and that can be pretty scary and difficult to sort through.

Books like these are usually written by a committee, often involving debate and compromise, whereas this book will give you the facts—the positives and the negatives—to help you weigh up the choices involved when you come to important decisions in your treatment journey.

One thing is certain: breast cancer is a complex area that I will try to break down and explain for you in plain English. I will also provide key results from the key breast cancer studies in easy-to-understand tables and graphs. If you are not a data person, just skip over these and read only the text. I don't like rushing patients, so I go slowly through all of their questions. Everybody is different, of course—some women like to be told what to do, others like a moderate amount of information, and still others like a lot. Some people like copies of our peer-reviewed publications. One size doesn't fit all.

Remember, it is important not to rush into treatment. You have plenty of time to find a team that will look after you in the best possible way both physically and emotionally. It's best to get the right treatment the first time, even a month after your diagnosis, than to be rushed into making the wrong decision.

I will use many garden and other analogies in this book. When you look at a flower, like a rose, you will see the complexities of the petals wrapping around each other. The health care system is also a complex maze, and in this book, using plain English examples often taken from nature, I will show you which turns to take so that you are taking control by always having the information you need at your fingertips.

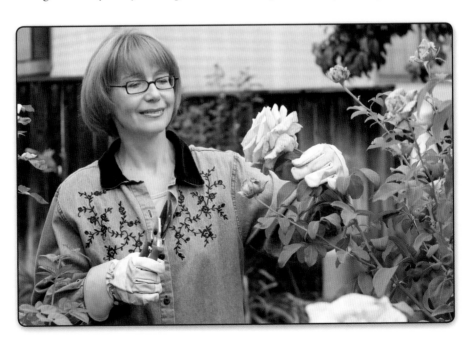

How to use this book

This book is not a textbook about breast cancer. It is a "behind the scenes" how-to book, designed to give you the key information you need at the 20 key "Control Points" on your path to survival. Flow charts for the "Control Points" are found at the beginning of each chapter and the complete set is shown at the back of the book.

Follow your possible paths and read the chapters that apply to your own situation. It's at these crossroads that you need the right information at the right time. In this book, there are three color themes used in the different parts as shown in the graphic below.

Part 1, in red, is the time to "stop" and take stock of the situation, rather than rush into a decision you may regret. Part 2 is in amber as a lot of "caution" is required in this part of your journey. Some big decisions need to be made that can affect the rest of your life. Part 3 is in green, which means to "proceed with care" and details information you need to have at your fingertips after your surgery and when all your treatment is over.

The book includes 15 real-life patient stories, 75 key web links, 96 figures and a reference list. Terms in the glossary are bolded when used in text for the first time.

Good luck in your journey, and I am sure that *Breast Cancer: Taking Control* will help you when life suddenly feels so out of control.

Part	Color	Action	Title	Taking Control	Control Points	Patient Stories
1	Red	STOP	Shock Control	Immediately after your diagnosis	2	7
2	Amber	CAUTION	Gaining Control	Before your surgery	6	2
3	Green	PROCEED WITH CARE	Maintaining Control	After your surgery	12	6

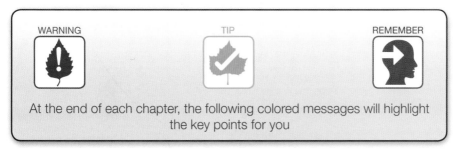

WARNING   TIP   REMEMBER

At the end of each chapter, the following colored messages will highlight the key points for you

Be treated as an individual

I constantly receive phone calls from friends, colleagues, or relatives who want advice about their individual situations. I decided that the only way to keep up with all of it was to write it down so that hopefully, others could learn from my experience. What I learned at Westmead Hospital and at Harvard University was critical—it taught me to delve into the medical literature and understand the natural history and the biology of breast cancer.

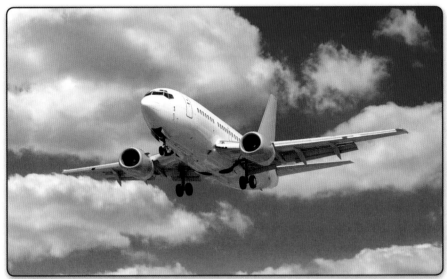

Figure 1: Find a pilot who knows how to deal with all weather conditions.

But there is no substitute for *experience*. I find that the difference between the good breast cancer doctors and the *really* good ones comes from treating lots of patients, particularly those who have a relapse or a difficult problem. Having treated fewer or simpler cases is like being a jet captain who has flown only in calm, sunny weather.

I like the older, gray-haired captains who have been around the world and flown in all sorts of conditions, even war zones. They know what to do when the going gets tough (Figure 1). Look at what Captain Chesley Sully Sullenberger faced when the plane he was flying crash-landed in the Hudson River. You don't land an airliner safely in the Hudson by working only in calm weather.

Most of our patients don't have a relapse, but working in a large referral center, I see many whose cancer has come back and I think, "If only the patient got the right treatment the first time." It's by understanding how, when, where, and why breast cancer comes back that we can effectively treat *you* as an *individual* patient.

The reason I stress the word "individual" is that with breast cancer, it's not as simple as using a recipe-book approach. I knew of one well known doctor who, by all accounts, had all the criteria for being a good breast cancer doctor. But when you looked closely at his figures, it was clear that nearly all of his patients had treatment by breast conservation (where the cancer is treated without a mastectomy, or breast removal). One of his colleagues had a nearly 100 percent mastectomy rate! These were two doctors in the same hospital treating the same mix of patients.

Iris's story on page 65 is a typical example of a surgeon's bias influencing treatment. For her, the right decision was to have a mastectomy.

I sent Iris back to her surgeon with what I thought was a diplomatically worded letter recommending a mastectomy. The surgeon called me the next day and essentially abused me for recommending such an outdated treatment.

A similar thing happened to me a few years later, when a general surgeon refused to perform a mastectomy for a patient who desperately needed it. Thankfully, that doesn't happen too often these days. I diplomatically wrote to him, saying that the patient wanted and needed a mastectomy and that I would be arranging it at my local hospital with an experienced breast surgeon.

Later, I'll tell you the real factors that influence whether a mastectomy is medically needed. Many surgeons used to recommend a mastectomy on very dubious grounds—sometimes based on medical misinformation—and sometimes they truly believed in their hearts that there was nothing better than the tried and tested "traditional mastectomy." That section includes many photos and a series of *key do's and don'ts* based on the best possible medical research.

"Why me?"

There are many causes of breast cancer, but the important things to note are that:

- There may be some causes of breast cancer that you can change. For example, you can stop taking a birth control pill or hormone replacement therapy.

- There may be factors associated with your breast cancer that you cannot change: for example, your family history or when you had your first child.

The best approach is not to be too hard on yourself. I see many patients who feel guilty because they wrongly perceive that a behavior in which they'd engaged may have caused their breast cancer. Sometimes in life, it depends on the roll of the dice, and we can't really explain why something happens to us. Sometimes, it may be for reasons that will take years to understand fully. It's important not to "rewind your tape," so to speak—to focus overly much on the past or the guilt and regrets that might come with it—and also not to "fast forward your tape"—to focus too much on the bewildering range of possibilities in the future. Rather, turn your energy toward the things that you can control.

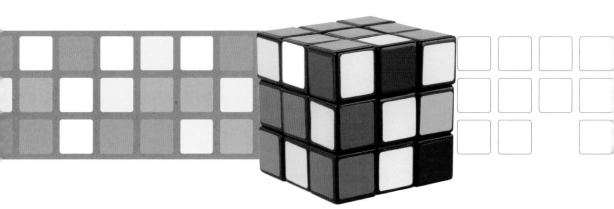

Figure 2: We really don't know exactly which factors cause breast cancer.

Some misguided reasons for breast cancer that are often stated in books or women's magazines include:

- My period started early
- I have always been overweight
- I started the pill when I was 16
- I took the pill for 20 years
- I've taken hormone replacement therapy (HRT or HT)
- My mother has had breast cancer
- It's all the stress in my life
- It's my job
- It's the hormones they feed to chickens
- It's the deodorant I've been using
- It's the bra I've been wearing.

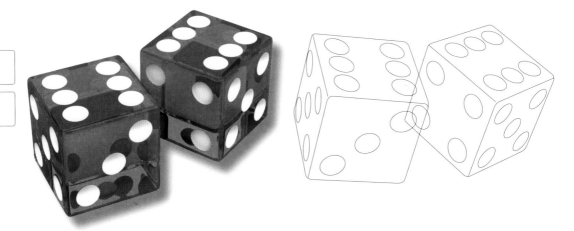

Figure 3: Sometimes it seems like it's just the roll of the dice.

Quite frankly, it's not that simple. The development of breast cancer is a complex Rubik's cube®.

You may look in one direction and see all the blue bits lining up, and one researcher may say that it's all genetic. You turn the cube around and some researcher states that it's all the hormones we've been using in Western society, and you turn the cube around again and see that maybe it's something that you've been doing with your diet, the pill, or HRT (Figure 2).

In summary, the dice have fallen in a particular way (Figure 3). You have breast cancer, and really shouldn't dwell too much on what might have caused it. If you have been taking HRT, then yes, consider stopping it, as it may have "fed" your cancer, particularly if your cancer is "**hormone positive**," or what we call "**estrogen receptor (ER) positive**."

I have treated many Seventh Day Adventists, vegetarians, and other people who have eaten well and exercised regularly. I have treated weight lifters, marathon runners, champion golfers, and tennis players, and they all got breast cancer with or without a family history. I have treated mothers who first had their baby when they were 17 and had eight children, and they still got breast cancer. I have treated women who have never taken the pill or HRT.

Fewer than five in one hundred women with breast cancer are thought to be linked in some way to alterations in the genes called **BRCA1 and BRCA2** (which is shorthand for breast cancer 1 and breast cancer 2). This is highest in families with a history of multiple members with breast cancer, where both breast and ovarian cancer are diagnosed in the same family, or in families with an Eastern European (Ashkenazi) Jewish background. However, not every woman in such families carries an alteration in BRCA1 or BRCA2, and not every cancer in such families is linked to alterations in these genes. If your doctor suspects a genetic link, he or she may see you and your family in a dedicated family history clinic and talk to you about arranging a blood test for the BRCA1 and BRCA2 gene changes or "mutations."

Breast cancer is common in Western society, but not that common. It is partly because we are getting older and are now facing more and more chronic diseases such as heart disease, diabetes, and cancers of all types. Incidentally, many forms of breast cancer have a better prognosis than a heart attack or indeed diabetes.

"Cancer" is just a word. Yes, it's a scary word, *but* it is a disease that can be beaten or a chronic disease that can be controlled, like diabetes. Just do your best to take control of the situation and keep reading.

Taking control means understanding the "garden" around you

I am not a gardener, but I find that most people have, at some time in their life, kept a garden or indoor plant or at least enjoyed walking through a public garden.

My attempts at gardening have always been a total failure, mainly because I immerse myself in breast cancer and not gardening. The last time my late father insisted on my having a vegetable garden, it was overridden by weeds. I had no time to look after and care for it and, quite frankly, I found it easier to go down to the local supermarket to buy fruit and vegetables than to try to care for a garden. However, my garden does illustrate how choices are made by all of us every day, and not just when we're struck with a serious illness.

One day, our home was hit by a wild storm. The fence fell over, and to my "horror," it landed right on my vegetable patch. I decided at this point that I had reached a "fork in the road," or a "Control Point."

This is what happens with breast cancer, not only in terms of treating the disease, but also in life decisions afterward.

When my fence fell, I had to decide:

- If I should immediately seek help from the neighbors, lift up the fence, and hold it up with some beams of wood to rescue the vegetable garden, or...

- If I should leave the fence on top of the vegetables, kill them off, and have a really good excuse to give my father for never having a vegetable garden again.

For me, it wasn't much of a choice. I decided to take control. I decided that I wanted no more vegetable gardens and preferred to either work on my research or, as my wife would say, "play with my computer."

I do, however, find that examples from nature help you understand the many choices you'll face, and I will use them throughout the book. I like to call these points "Control Points" because they are a combination of important steps you need to take at the right time—important decisions and choices—*taking control* of these decisions by having the right information.

For me, taking control of the decision to leave the fence on the vegetables gave me freedom in some ways—I made the decision based on information, it was right for me, and it allowed me to go down another path without having the mental pain of worrying about weeding or getting results I really didn't need.

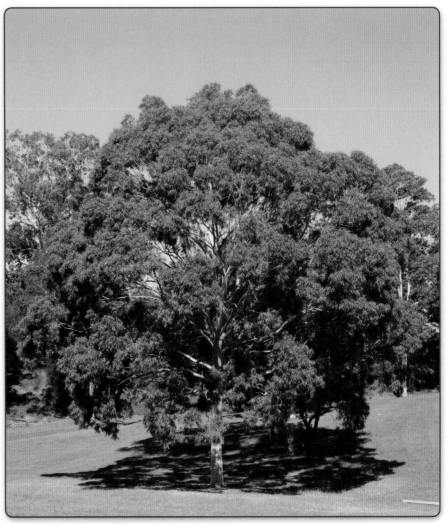

Figure 4: An Australian gum tree.

Before I give you the 20 essential Control Points you need to navigate not only your new diagnosis but also an often complex health system, I will talk a little about how breast cancer starts and what it looks like under a microscope. From there I will give you the 20 Control Points you need to think about to ensure that you get the best possible care.

The breast, believe it or not, is not unlike our Australian gum tree (Figure 4). I don't know the scientific name of the gum tree, despite the fact that Peter, whom I walk with two to three times a week, regularly points them out. Unfortunately, the name goes in one ear and out the other. At times, it's a bit like receiving medical information when Peter tells me the scientific names of plants.

The trunk at the base of the plant is like the large ducts near the nipple. As we move toward the back of the breast and toward the skin, there are smaller and smaller branches and then smaller and smaller twigs. Where the twigs and the leaves meet, this is known as the **terminal duct lobular unit**. We've been told for years by various pathologists that this is where breast cancer actually begins. It is probably true in most cases. For some reason, the area where the leaf joins the twig becomes unstable, and the cells can change.

The picture below shows a breast, the **ducts** (the small pipes that carry milk from the breast glands), and the breast **glands** (where the milk is produced during lactation). The leaves are the **lobules** where milk is produced, and the branches are the ducts (Figure 5).

It is hard to know what makes the cells change. What you need to know at the moment is that if you obtain a little garden saw and cut through one of these ducts, you would normally see a hollow tube with a single lining of cells. Figure 6 shows how a branch or duct looks when cut through.

With time, the cells can become heaped up. When the cells heap up a bit more, this is called **hyperplasia**, which means "too many cells." When the heaped-up cells don't look typical, this is called **atypia**, meaning not typical or not normal (Figure 6).

It's the last two diagrams in Figure 6 that I really want you to concentrate on for now. If the cells begin to look like cancer cells and are still confined within the duct, it's called **ductal carcinoma in situ**, or **DCIS**. I call this "pre-cancer" because the cells have not yet invaded through the duct, and I often explain this as a pipe that is very strong on the outside but contains some rust on the inside that has not yet penetrated the surface of the pipe.

If you have been diagnosed with **invasive carcinoma**, the cancer has penetrated through the pipe—burst through the duct wall. This is also referred to as invasive ductal carcinoma or **infiltrating ductal carcinoma**, which means essentially the same thing—that there is an invasive carcinoma or you have a diagnosis of breast cancer.

Cancer cells can spread via small vessels, called **lymphatics**, that carry fluid called **lymph** all around our body, including in the breast. Lymphatics are connected to **lymph glands** or nodes, which are found in the armpit (also known as the **axilla**) and around the breastbone (the **sternum**) and collarbone (the **clavicle**). The **lymphatic system** is part of the immune system, which helps to fight infection and can stop cancer cells in the glands.

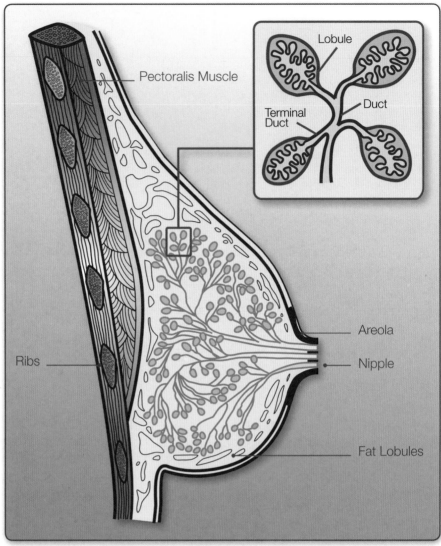

Figure 5: Cross-section of the breast.

Now that you've been told you have breast cancer, it is important to understand clearly what needs to be done. I'd like to go back to my garden example. Except this time, there are four garden patches.

The garden patches are like the different **stages** in breast cancer (Figure 7).

- The first garden patch has a rose bush, and under this rose, there is a weed. Let's assume this weed is your breast cancer and the rose bush is your breast. This is called "stage 1."

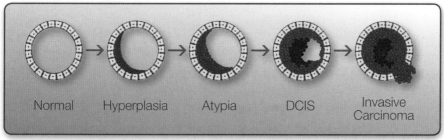

Figure 6: Cross-section of a breast duct going from normal to invasive carcinoma.

- The next garden patch looks okay, and there are no weeds in it. This next stage is like your "axilla" or armpit. If the weed or the cancer goes to this next garden patch, it is called "stage 2."

- A weed that spreads from under the rose bush to the next patch and the one after is like a large cancer that is very advanced in the breast and gland areas, which we call "stage 3."

- A weed that affects a faraway part of the garden is like a cancer that affects different parts of the body, such as the liver or lungs, and is called "stage 4."

It's important to map out what's going on—not only what type of cancer you have but also how far it has travelled. Not having information can be very isolating at times (Figure 8).

Understanding your type of breast cancer

The pathologist will call the invasive carcinomas by different names depending on the pattern of the invasion. The most common type of cancer is an invasive ductal carcinoma (Figure 9).

Invasive lobular carcinoma is the second most common type of invasive cancer. It starts off in the lobules, or "leaves," and has a distinctive pattern (Figure 10). The pathology report may say "single file" because the cells are usually round, uniform in appearance, and lined up as if walking in a line. The unusual thing about lobular cancer is that it does not cause any reaction in the normal tissue. Ductal carcinoma, for example, can cause scarring, which in turn can cause drawing in of the nipple or dimpling of the skin.

Lobular carcinomas, on the other hand, are what I call "sneaky" carcinomas. They tend to cause less reaction and thus often go undetected for longer.

The good news about lobular cancers is that they tend to be hormone positive or, **estrogen receptor positive**, opening them up to more treatment options.

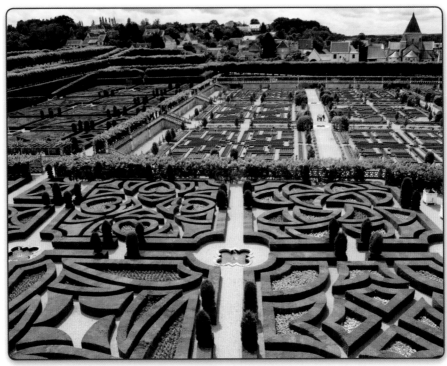

Figure 7: There are four stages of breast cancer, like four garden patches.

However, lobular cancers are often hard to detect on a mammogram. So, if you are worried at any time about your breast and the mammogram is normal, insist on an **ultrasound** or biopsy to be sure.

An invasive **tubular carcinoma** means that it contains a lot of little tubules (little pipes that look like the normal ducts). Tubular carcinomas are generally discovered through breast screening in very early stages and have an exceptionally good prognosis (Figure 11). **Mucinous carcinomas** have a lot of mucus, which floats around the ducts and lobules when the pathologist looks at it through the microscope (Figure 12). **Medullary carcinoma** is also a special type of infiltrating breast cancer that is noted by its well defined edge between the tumor and the surrounding normal tissue. It also has some other special features, including the large size of the cancer cells and the presence of immune system cells called lymphocytes at the edges of the tumor. The outlook (prognosis) for this kind of breast cancer is generally better than for the more common types of invasive breast cancer.

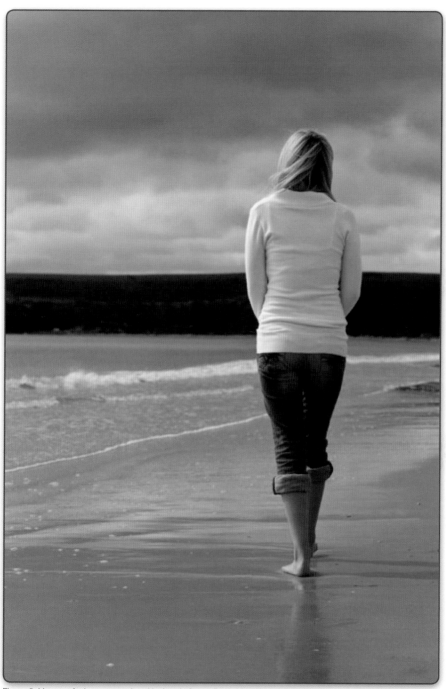

Figure 8: You can feel very scared and isolated after a diagnosis of breast cancer.

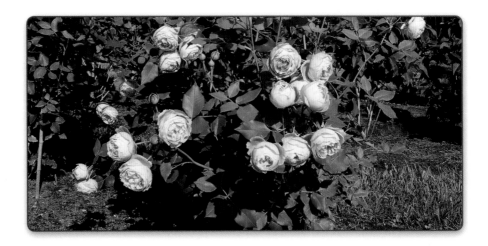

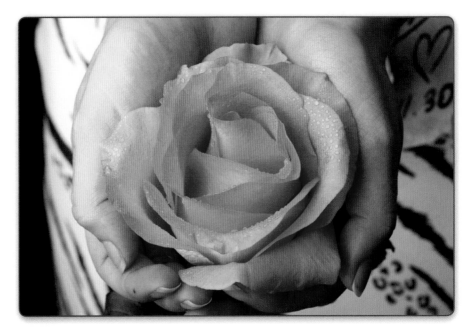

True medullary carcinoma is quite rare. These cancers, originally called "atypical medullary carcinoma" because of the presence of immune cells, are now thought to be associated with a genetic type of breast cancer linked to the BRCA1-affected gene. These tumors tend to be **"triple negative"** and are also called "basal-like," and may have a slightly worse prognosis than other cancers.

The different types of breast cancer, in general, are not that important, since both your treatment and prognosis are governed by how big a cancer is when it's first discovered and whether or not it has spread to the lymph glands under your armpit.

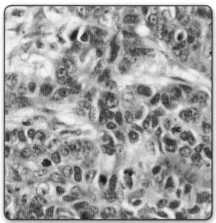

Figure 9: Invasive ductal carcinoma as seen under a microscope.

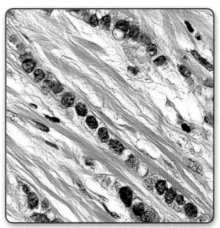

Figure 10: Invasive lobular carcinomas have small cells that line up in a row.

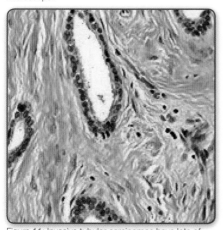

Figure 11: Invasive tubular carcinomas have lots of tubules, like normal ducts of the breast.

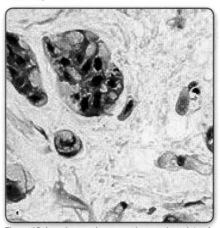

Figure 12: Invasive mucinous carcinomas have lots of mucus surrounding the cells.

Later, in Control Point #11, I will explain the difference between stage and **grade**. Briefly though, to use my garden example, stage is how far along the four garden patches a weed has travelled (from 1 to 4). Grade actually describes the weed itself. A grade 1 tumor is more ordered and less likely to spread. It's a bit like a broad leaf weed in the garden, with very little seed, and tends never to come back when you pull it out. A grade 3 tumor, on the other hand, divides more quickly and looks less ordered and more haphazard under the microscope. It's a bit like one of those annoying onion weeds that have a tendency to come back after you remove them.

What is really important is to take control of the situation by understanding key points of your treatment, or what some people call "your journey." Some decisions and steps need to take place before any surgery (Part 2), and some can only take place after your surgery (Part 3). I'll discuss them all.

PART 1

"SHOCK CONTROL"

TAKING CONTROL IMMEDIATELY
AFTER DIAGNOSIS

Jenny's Story

Jenny worked in public service, and she'd known for about two months that she had a lump in her left breast. She was very scared, and especially afraid to go have it checked out. After she was told she had breast cancer by her general practitioner, she was referred to a general surgeon, but decided to do a bit of research first.

When she came and saw our team, she told me about her research. She said, "Everything pointed to you guys." She did a search of breast cancer articles in the media and saw which doctors were giving expert opinions in the leading daily newspaper; she found colleagues at work who had had treatment; she called the cancer help line for advice.

"When my mum's bingo group recommended you as well," she said, "I knew this was the place to come."

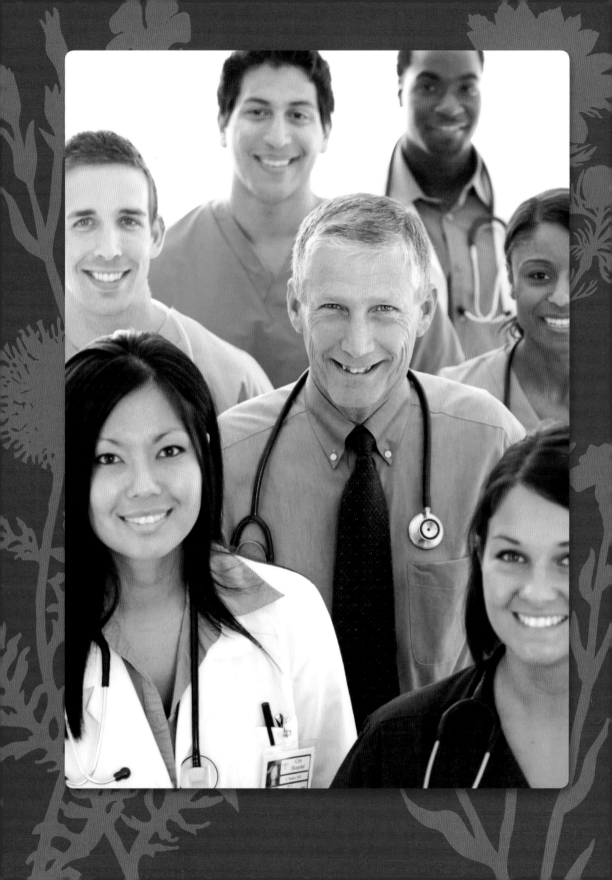

Control Point 1

How Do I Find the Right Treatment Team?

Control Point #1

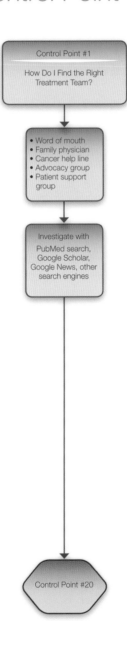

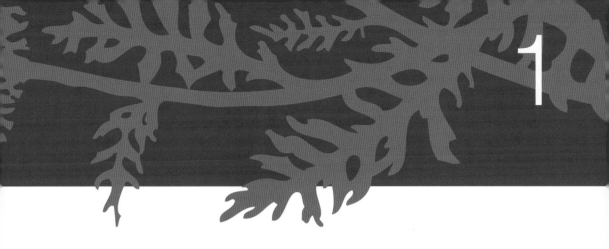

How Do I Find the Right Treatment Team?

It pays to do some research about your doctors

It's very scary when you find out you have breast cancer. You may have found a lump or had an abnormal **mammogram** and then a **biopsy**. Your whole life stops; nothing else matters all of a sudden. Your work takes second priority, you often can't hear what is going on around you, and a lot of the information you receive from doctors, nurses and well-meaning friends and relatives often goes in one ear and out the other. You lose control, and decisions may be made for you in a hurry.

Believe me, at this point, there are times when it seems like a mountain has just landed on the road you're traveling on and you simply can't climb over it: lots of doctors; waiting rooms; information; searching the web and obtaining information from various support groups, help lines, or outdated books in your local library.

I want to hold you by the hand and show you the path to climb this mountain and get to the other side.

I hope that when you were told about your breast cancer, you had somebody with you. It is particularly hard being told on your own. Take somebody with you whenever you're reaching key crossroads, when you need to make a choice, or when you're receiving important results such as your pathology reports after your surgery. Give your support person this book to read, as well, so they also have the knowledge to help you.

Knowledge helps you gain control by learning nearly as much as your doctor about breast cancer in these vital first weeks after your diagnosis. These are the critical steps to take on day one to regain some control over your situation:

- Remember that breast cancer is not a "medical emergency"—a few extra days to ensure that you get the right information and treatment won't harm you

- Understand your choices and don't get rushed into a decision you don't feel comfortable about. Find the best option for your own individual situation.

- Find a doctor who can deliver that option safely and efficiently without significant waiting times

- Take notes, ask your support person to be a note-taker, or take a tape recorder with you

- Ask for a copy of letters or other correspondence doctors send to each other

- Keep a copy of all your test results and correspondence in ascending chronological order in one of those folders with lots of clear plastic sheets

- Keep a copy of details of your insurance company, policy number, contact telephone numbers, health care cards, and a log of important dates including your consultations, dates of surgery, when you started and finished radiation therapy, chemotherapy or hormonal treatment

- Write your telephone number on all your X-rays, as they often get lost

- Inquire about cancer support groups and consider keeping a journal or blog of your thoughts, experiences and feelings

- See if your team includes a breast care nurse, who is usually more accessible than the doctor, and ask for his or her business card or best contact number

- Ask for a business card from all the professionals you meet

- Better still, find a doctor who works in a team—a **surgeon**, a **radiation oncologist**, and a **medical oncologist**. The team should work closely with other specialists, such as a **plastic surgeon** and a geneticist, and have access to expert nurses and other allied health staff.

- If you live outside a large city, it is of course harder to see the whole team before your surgery. Seek an opinion from a surgeon who has networks with a cancer center, or if you can afford the time, money, extra stress, and inconvenience of leaving your home, seek a second opinion.

- Be prepared to take control of your destiny, particularly during follow-up, as most doctors don't have the time to provide you the emotional support you need.

Understand the "aerial view" of your treatment journey by reading the "Control Points" flow charts at the start of each chapter, and at the end of the book. Refer back to these frequently when you come to important steps or decision points.

This should not turn into a doctor-bashing exercise. Rather, it's about you understanding the medical aspects of the disease, what is possible and what is not possible, and what treatments can and cannot be given safely in a particular situation. Do your research, but don't go overboard. Be particularly guided by your family doctor, who knows you and your medical history.

Do a Google search of the doctor to whom you've been referred. See what articles he or she has written. This will give you a guide to a doctor's specific interests and expertise and may give you a clue to whether he or she works as part of a team. One quick way of doing this is via **Google Scholar**. Go to www.Google.com and click "more," then find the Google Scholar link in the drop-down menu. To find some of my articles, type in "John Boyages" with the quotation marks, as this gives a more exact search (Figure 13). Do the same thing in Google and type in your doctor's name in quotation marks. Here is what happens; Google Scholar found 145 articles, and when I clicked on "Recent articles," it found 52. It doesn't pick them all up.

Here is another way to do a search of your doctor's publications that is probably more accurate. **PubMed** was developed at the National Library of Medicine, located at the US National Institutes of Health (NIH). It indexes all of the journals in MEDLINE and many other citations. **MEDLINE** contains citations from 1950 to the present, with a focus on the biomedical sciences. Approximately 5,200 journals published in the US and more than 80 other countries have been selected and are currently indexed for MEDLINE, and are therefore included in PubMed. To start a PubMed search, type in the following (Figure 14):

www.ncbi.nlm.nih.gov/sites/entrez

Now press "Search" (to the right of where you entered the author's name) and see what happens (Figure 15). Today's search shows that I have 96 publications indexed in PubMed. Remember, this is not all of an individual's publications, as some journals are not indexed in MEDLINE or PubMed, particularly those outside the US, but it does give you a guide on what (and when) they have published.

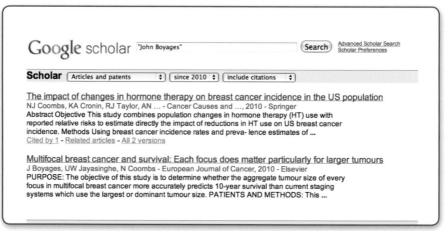

Figure 13: A Google Scholar search is a good way to start investigating your doctor.

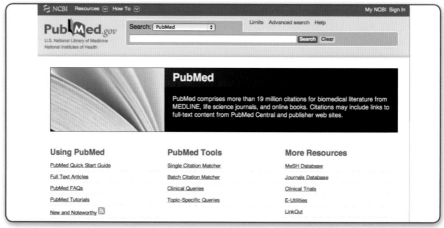

Figure 14: A PubMed search on your doctor will show you most of their published work.

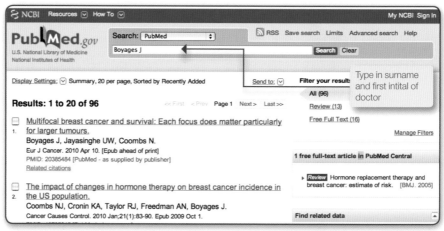

Figure 15: The results of a PubMed search indicate the research interests of your doctor.

Judith's Story

My consultation with my GP helped me to define the parameters of my search initially. I would look for someone who was a specialist in breast surgery, rather than a general surgeon who did some breast surgery. I would look for someone who was not too young and not too old—probably late forties to fifties—old enough to have gained a lot of experience but not someone who was looking toward retirement and might not be in touch with the latest research and techniques.

I needed someone who was not only good at surgery, but who would also listen to me and treat me as an individual. In order to find a surgeon who met my needs, I spoke to several doctors who are friends or family, asking for their recommendations and who they would go to or send a family member to for breast surgery in Sydney. I also spoke to several women who had had breast surgery, asking about their opinions of their doctors. I was now looking for a person who was part of a multidisciplinary team.

I wanted doctors who would talk to me, listen to me, and talk to each other about me. By now, I had several doctors, scientists, and other health professionals asking around on my behalf, and their recommendations were starting to come in. We were also praying. My journal at the time says, "I am praying that God will make my path plain, as the Bible says. We will just keep gathering information and praying and waiting until it is clear which is the path God wants me to take."

I phoned the "A," "B," "C," and "D" hospitals to get information about how their teams worked together. It seemed clear that "D" was the only true team. The others met weekly or less often, but were basically separate clinicians who referred their patients to each other. One of the most useful things to me in finding a team was the approachability of the team I ended up with.

In those first few days before surgery, my choice was confirmed over and over. Their names continued to come in as recommendations from other patients and my doctor friends, and both Owen and John were willing to talk to me on the phone to answer my questions about what type of surgery I should have. That level of approachability is very rare. I had found what I was looking for—a team who treated me as an individual rather than a body with breast cancer, listened to me, talked to me, talked to each other, were at the top of their profession in the eyes of their peers, and their patients couldn't speak highly enough of them. Neither can I.

But please remember that this is only a guide. There are some really fabulous doctors who are just busy being good doctors and attending education updates at conferences who do not have the time or writing skills required to publish. Some doctors who are very prolific in publications may not necessarily be the best technical surgeons or best communicators. Do your research, but keep it in perspective. You need a doctor who can look after you well and keep up with the latest information, and who is prepared to listen to *your* needs.

In some countries, there are directories of doctors. In Australia, the Breast Cancer Action Group NSW developed the national Breast Cancer Directory with information about individual surgeons, radiation oncologists, and medical oncologists (Breast Cancer Action Group NSW 2002). One patient I treated, simply asked the radiologist who biopsied the abnormaility in her breast, who he'd take his wife to, if she was diagnosed with breast cancer.

Often, your national cancer organization is aware of any available directories. In the US, consider going to an NCI (National Cancer Institute)-designated cancer center or a center affiliated with a university medical school. There are also many community cancer programs where doctors are part of a **multidisciplinary team** that includes surgeons, oncologists, radiologists, breast care nurses, and many other team members. If you're not comfortable with your doctor or team, seek a second opinion. The American Cancer Society may be able to help find you a team that will suit your circumstances. They can be contacted at 1-800-ACS-2345. They can also help with support groups. In Australia, the Cancer Council helpline can be contacted at 13-11-20.

Don't forget to encourage at least one designated friend or family member to read this book and attend your appointments with you. It's quite easy to "go blank" during a consultation and not really hear what is being said when you're still in a state of shock.

Also, if you are in Australia, the Breast Cancer Network Australia has some good information that can support you at the point of diagnosis, including their "My Journey Kit," which you can order by calling 1300 785 562 or by visiting:

www.bcna.org.au/content/view/16/20/

This free kit provides an information guide, a personal journal where you can record important information about your cancer and its treatment, and a satchel to store copies of test results, the information guide, and anything else you want to save. It's a great resource and I really encourage you to get one.

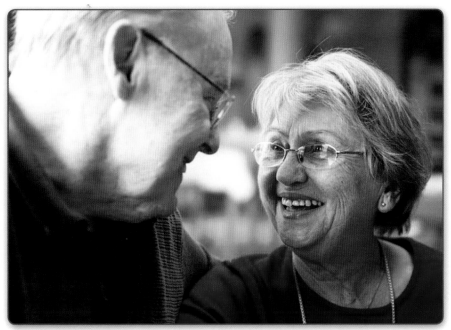
Figure 16: Remember that most people beat breast cancer, and life will start to improve again.

What's really important at this point is family and friends (Figure 16). At the point of diagnosis, most women feel they are going to die, but the reality is that *most women beat breast cancer*. I've been continuously impressed by the rapid growth of knowledge in the field of genetics, as well as the discovery of better "targeted" therapies, chemotherapy and **radiation therapy**, which have already made a difference in improving the cure rates from breast cancer.

CONTROL POINT #1– HOW DO I FIND THE RIGHT TREATMENT TEAM?

WARNING Understand your choices and don't get rushed into a decision you don't feel comfortable about.

TIP Take a few extra days to find the right team. Find a doctor who works in a team that includes a surgeon, a radiation oncologist, and a medical oncologist.

REMEMBER Breast cancer is not a medical emergency. It pays to do some research about your doctors.

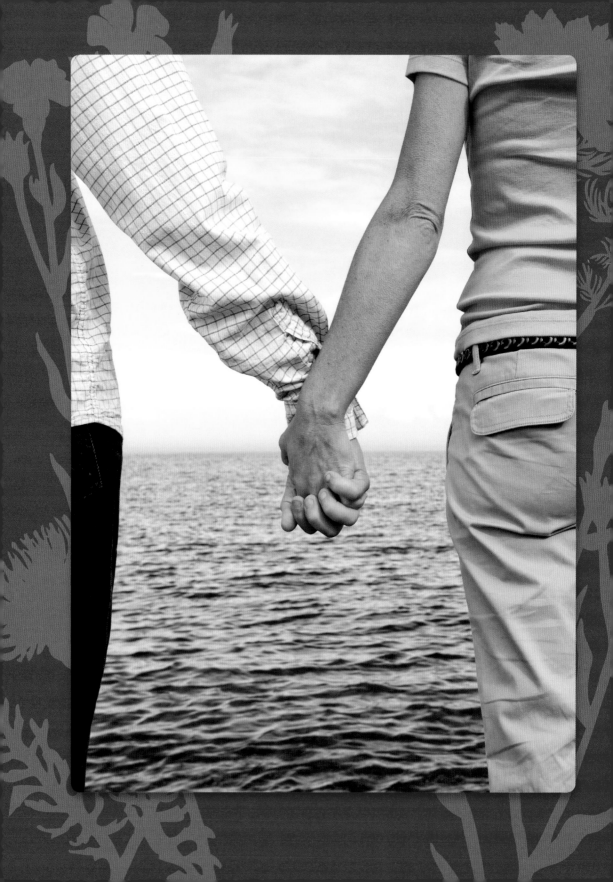

Control Point 2

How Do I Cope with My
Family and Friends?

Control Point #2

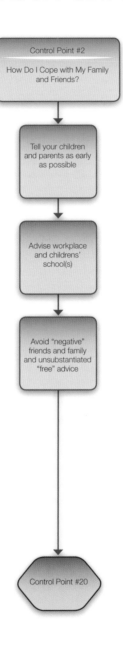

2

How Do I Cope with My Family and Friends?

Breaking your news to others

There is absolutely no doubt that this is a tough call. Who do you tell? What can you say? When do you say something? How do you tell someone else that "I have breast cancer"? There's no right way of doing this. "I've been to the doctor today and they said I might (or do) have breast cancer." Keep it short and sweet, and most people will give you a hug or say, "I'm really sorry to hear that." Have lots of tissues around at this time. It's better to let the tears out—it's very therapeutic. I worry about women who can't cry either privately or with others. It's good for you to have the catharsis of crying out your emotions. And remember that while there are certainly some storm clouds around, most clouds have a silver lining, and some good nearly always comes out of this illness (Figure 17).

Sit down, have a glass of wine or your favorite drink, and just regroup. You have been hurt by the diagnosis, shocked and scared, but you're still alive and can take action to fight this disease. It's hard to believe. Most of my patients say, "I can't believe I have breast cancer," or "It can't be happening to me."

Talk to your partner, husband, relative, or best friend and let them know what's going on. You don't have to bear the shock of your diagnosis alone.

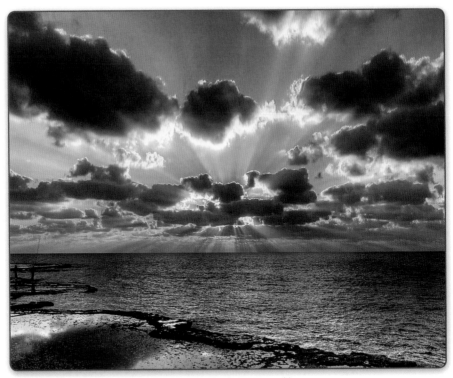

Figure 17: Always look for a silver lining when storm clouds are approaching.

If you have children, talk to them about your disease. A good resource is at the following website from the United Kingdom (UK):

www.breastcancercare.org.uk/server/show/nav.347

Talk to your family, preferably in person. This is often difficult, and some family members and friends really don't know what to say. Some people, in fact, may stop calling you. This can hurt, but don't be too hard on them—it's often just a reaction to their own mortality, or they may not want to upset you or get in your way while you're on treatment.

Telling your children

Ensure open communication. Children usually know something is going on (Figure 18). They can see it in your face. Sit down with them after you've seen the doctor and tell them you need to investigate your breast lump or abnormality on your mammogram, and things will be all right after you have your treatment. Nobody knows what's around the corner for any of us, so trying to give hope to your children is important to everyone's sense of wellbeing.

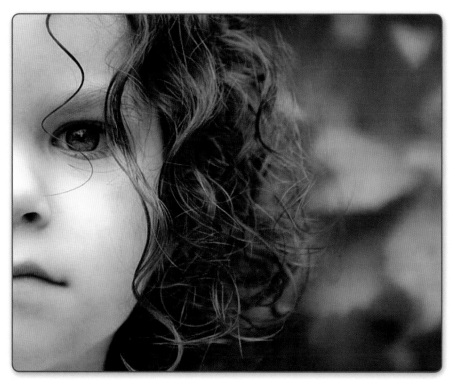
Figure 18: Talking to your children is hard but essential.

Children are very intuitive, and they know when something is wrong. The problem with not telling them you have breast cancer is that they may instead think that you're having marriage difficulties or that they're a part of the problem, and they won't realize that you're only trying to protect them.

They will certainly pick up on the whispered conversations between adults, so at some point, it's important to sit down with them. It's better to do this as a group so they can all get the same amount of information at the same time. Before talking with your children, talk with your doctor or your breast care nurse and, of course, with your partner to decide what you will and will not say. Perhaps even practice the wording that you'll use. I find that the best approach is to keep things very simple and just see what questions your children ask.

If the tumor is undiagnosed, I suggest using the word "lump." You might want to say, "Mommy has a lump in her breast." Then say, "The doctors want to do a biopsy, or take a sample, or remove it." It's always important to follow that up by saying, "Mommy will be all right."

The word "cancer" is out there today in the media. There are many celebrities who have had cancer and survived, and there are others, of course, whose cancer came back.

Once you know that you are dealing with cancer, you or your partner can say something like, "Mommy does have breast cancer. She's going to be all right, but will need extra treatment." Or, "I will lose my hair with the treatment but it will grow back." Or, "I will need to go to the hospital every day to have a special treatment to stop the cancer from coming back."

Each child behaves differently. Some become very quiet, others become more cuddly and clingy and may want to sleep in bed with you, and others may have behavioral problems. Give them opportunities to talk about your cancer and your treatment— even with other friends or relatives or schoolmates.

Speak to the school counselor so they'll be more understanding if your child finds it difficult to concentrate at school. Of course you have to maintain normal discipline and try to keep the family together as much as possible during what may be a very difficult treatment program, but always keep them informed.

It's important to continue your child's routine and still drive them to and from school, take them to activities, and spend time with them. Keeping up the routine as much as practically possible is very comforting and reassuring to them. It can be hard when you feel tired from your treatments. Perhaps spend time with them doing less strenuous activities such as watching television, reading a book, or watching one of their favorite movies. Sometimes, depending on the type of surgery you've had, showing them your scar may be important in the healing process.

Some children come along to radiation therapy treatments. Most staff members are happy to watch the kids while you're having your treatment, and this tends to demystify the whole situation for the children.

With very young children, it's important that they realize that the cancer is not their fault. I remember an older gentleman who said that his mother had died of breast cancer and that he bumped her breast as a teenager. He asked me if he could have caused the cancer. He was probably feeling guilty for years for something he absolutely didn't cause.

In summary, a parent's dilemma is the balance between protecting the child versus enabling understanding. Children need information to be truthful yet hopeful, and they need reassurance about ongoing love and stability, whatever the outcome.

Talking with and managing teenagers

Teenagers are probably the hardest group to deal with, particularly boys. They can go quiet and just ignore the whole situation. You may find this quite disturbing, but just try to give them time, and some hugs, and tell them you're going to be all right.

Make sure you still have time to go to their sports or activities and keep up their routine. Teenage boys may find the whole thing embarrassing. They may feel torn between being supportive, and wanting to be out with their friends and stay cool and rebellious. Although this can be difficult, it's best to keep the conversation light or get the boy's father or a close friend or mentor to talk to him about your diagnosis.

Teenage girls may become anxious because they feel they will automatically get breast cancer too. It's important to reassure them that most breast cancers do not occur in people who have a family history of the disease. Don't be too hard on your teenagers. Give them some space and keep answering their questions.

But remember, it's not enough to talk to them once and then not talk to them again about the situation. Tell them when there has been a change in your treatment plan, when things go right, or if things don't go as well as expected.

It is also important not to put too much "guilt" onto teenagers, for example, by expecting them to clean up their room when they've never cleaned their room before. Kids want you "back to normal" as quickly as possible, and I find that it's important for you as well to be "back to normal" as quickly as possible after your diagnosis. This includes going to work.

Dealing with your partner

Many male (or female) partners will be shocked by their loved one's diagnosis of breast cancer.

Men commonly have difficulty concentrating; they can't sleep, and experience feelings of loss and sadness (Figure 19). Traditionally, men are the "protectors," and suddenly they're facing a challenge in which they often feel helpless and sometimes very isolated. It is a problem they can't just go out and "fix."

Because breast cancer is life threatening, both women and their partners often fear death from the disease. Yet many men feel they cannot mention this fear because saying so might be "negative."

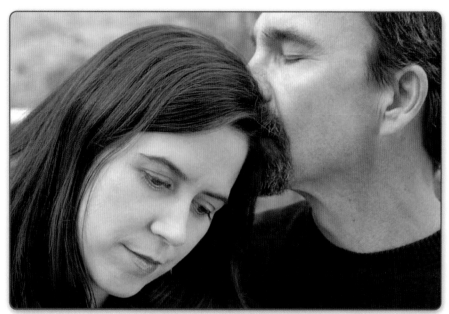
Figure 19: Some men find it really hard to cope when their partner is diagnosed with breast cancer.

Many men are challenged by parental, employment, domestic, and financial changes that come about when a woman is diagnosed with breast cancer. The distress and practical support needs of caretakers are frequently overlooked and need to be acknowledged, particularly because caretakers have to deal with their own response and distress as well as yours.

I recently treated a woman whose husband lost his job because he was spending so much time with her, taking her to medical and test appointments. Life can be very cruel at times.

Some men rise to the occasion and provide outstanding support, while others get "too involved" and overprotective, which can be frustrating. I have also seen men just walk out on their partners. So, it's critical to keep communicating with each other during this difficult time.

It's best to read this section together with your partner and try at all times to talk about your mutual feelings. This is often not a natural thing for males to do, so women, who are generally more experienced at sharing their feelings, should try to be patient with them.

Men may be embarrassed to talk about your diagnosis at work. In some cultures, it may bring "shame" to the family. In others, the woman is expected to keep doing everything "as normal" around the house, at work, and in the bedroom!

It can be very, very hard, but most women show enormous strength and get through this difficult post-diagnosis phase. Men also fear asking for attention at a time when they believe their partner or loved one should be the focus of attention. Men who fail to speak out or seek emotional support may experience higher levels of distress.

But remember, everyone gets through this phase. Treatment always finishes, appointments stop, and it's very important that life goes on, including intimacy and short escapes. Plan little breaks away—weekend vacations (even one night away), without the children—and keep on talking with each other.

Dealing with friends

All of us have different levels of friendships. We may have a very close friend with whom we can express our true thoughts and feelings. Have a "cuppa" with your best friend and tell him or her what's going on.

If friends stop calling you, either ignore them or give them a call and say, "You've probably heard that I've been diagnosed with breast cancer. I'm going to be all right and I'd be very grateful if you could pop in and see me or run an errand or prepare a meal." This may break the ice, or you may decide to leave friends alone for the moment if they don't call you.

Another option is just to be upfront about the diagnosis and leave it there, and see who emerges to offer a helping hand. Often, there'll be new friends made at this time. It's another important chapter of your life, and just as you made new friends when your children started school or you started a new job, you will find new friends who understand your journey with breast cancer.

Some of my patients have friends that always seem to upset them or say the wrong thing. They may be giving "free advice" and talking to you about the latest herb, potion, or lotion that may help with your breast cancer. Listen to them, but don't become too engaged with this behavior.

I particularly worry about the "friends" who tell you of other patients who died of breast cancer and link their death to a particular treatment they may or may not have had, such as breast conservation or a mastectomy, when in fact it had no relevance to their treatment at all from a medical or scientific perspective. (See "Harold's" story below.) Thank your friends for their advice. Maybe say, "I feel a bit overwhelmed by all the advice I'm getting at the moment, but thank you anyway. For now, I'm going to follow my doctor's advice."

Anne's Story

I recently spoke with Anne, who was planning to quit her job. She had been working in sales for over 20 years and as a sales manager more recently. She thought she should resign. When I inquired why, she said, "I'm just finding it stressful trying to cope with my breast cancer and holding down a full-time job and managing people at the same time."

There were lots of tears, and I could see that Anne was really hurting about losing her job. I replied, "You look like the sort of person who enjoys working with customers and really helping them." I said to her, "It's hopeless when we improve and they throw us into management and you have to leave what you like doing. It's like the good teacher who gets promoted to the principal of the school and gets away from face-to-face teaching. Have you thought about going back to the shop floor and still getting paid for what you like doing?" Breast cancer allows a time for reflection and possible change for the better.

Gloria's Story

Gloria was a young mom who did not tell her children that she had breast cancer until three months before she died. She was trying to protect them, of course.

I asked her to write a letter to each of them, talking about her feelings and why she couldn't tell them earlier. They were all aged ten or younger, but they knew something was going on. She went through chemotherapy, lost her hair, and wore wigs at all times to hide her condition.

I was very worried about her reaction, but obviously had to support her way of dealing with it. She had a very, very supportive husband. Gloria was a very brave woman, but I felt helpless with her way of dealing with the cancer. Keep communicating with the people closest to you whenever possible.

Harold's Story

One of our "friends," "Gerard," kept calling and giving us "advice." He was concerned that Ruth had chosen to have breast conservation and not a mastectomy.

Gerard knew two work colleagues whose wives had died of cancer that had spread to their bones, and both hadn't had a mastectomy.

Ruth was getting anxious about all this, and in the end, I gave Gerard a call and said, "Look, I really appreciate the care you are showing to Ruth, but she is finding your stories of your two friends at work a bit scary.

"Would you mind backing off a little in terms of medical advice, as Ruth really needs to have confidence in her decisions." Gerard stopped calling after that.

But I really thought I had to stand up to him, although it was very, very difficult.

Tania's Story

Tania worked in an office a short walk from one of our hospitals. She was having daily radiation treatment, which took about half an hour each day, and no chemotherapy.

Her treatment was going well, and apart from some minor skin reddening, there were no other side effects.

I encouraged her to work throughout her treatment. She saw me for a check-up and was very upset because the nurse in the hospital said to her that she was "stupid for working." Unbelievable!

Dealing with your employer

The reality is that many of my patients continue to work while having radiation therapy and even chemotherapy. At the outset, you really don't know how you will feel or react. Don't throw in your job just because you have breast cancer.

Everyone finds losing his or her hair very, very traumatic. It can be particularly hard for women who are receptionists or in other customer service roles that are on the front line.

The decision to stop working will depend on lots of factors, including where you live, where you work, where your treatment is to be undertaken, and the complexity of your treatment. Usually, you will be off work for about four to six weeks after your surgery, but you can get back to work after you start radiation or perhaps after your first dose of chemotherapy, once you know how you'll cope with any side effects.

I find that people who stay at work often cope much better than they would sitting at home and just staring at the walls. But if you'd prefer to take sick leave and can afford to stop work for a little while, you now have the perfect excuse to do so.

This is why you need to take control and know what's best for you, because you may get conflicting advice. Sometimes, it's from trainees who don't have much experience; sometimes, it's from doctors or other health professionals; and, of course, the Internet can be a challenge with the vast range of information and alternative treatments and solutions you can find there. Take care with the Internet, and look at some of the sites I recommend at the back of this book.

Breast cancer is often a good reason to change aspects of your life or work you don't particularly like for the better. Consider working part time before resigning, or try to take some paid or unpaid leave. If you really hate your job, maybe this is the time to move on! Plan a vacation after your treatment (Figure 20).

Most of my patients find they can usually work during radiation therapy by having their treatment first thing in the morning or by taking the last appointment in the afternoon. You may need to get to bed a little earlier because radiation therapy can cause some tiredness, but not enough to interrupt your normal routine or stop you from working.

If you need chemotherapy, some women find it's often best on a Friday so that you have the weekend to recover and get back to work the following week. Of course, everyone is different, and the important point is to take your time to work out what's best for you. Again don't rush this decision.

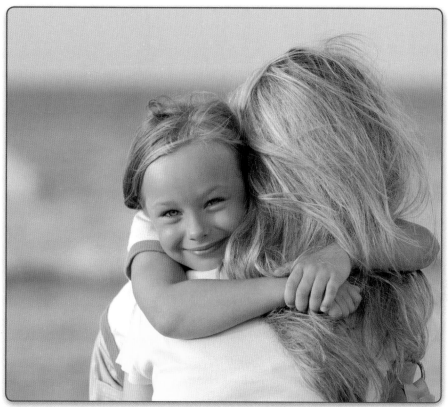

Figure 20: Life usually gets better once your treatment ends. Plan a vacation.

Control Point #2 – HOW DO I COPE WITH MY FAMILY AND FRIENDS?

WARNING

Avoiding telling your close family, especially your children, about your diagnosis will only add to your stress. Tell them sooner rather than later.

TIP

Breast cancer is often the perfect excuse to change aspects of your life or work you don't particularly like for the better.

REMEMBER

While there are certainly some storm clouds around, most clouds have a silver lining, and some good nearly always comes out of this illness.

PART 2

"GAINING CONTROL"

TAKING CONTROL BEFORE YOUR SURGERY

Iris's Story

Iris was in her 70s and was referred to me for an opinion about radiation therapy. Her surgeon wanted me to talk to her about radiation before she had her breast conserving surgery. She had a largish tumor in the upper, outer part of the breast and a gland involved in the armpit.

I asked her about her social circumstances, particularly because she had come alone and was a widow (her husband had passed away six months earlier). I asked her how she traveled to see me, because she lived at least 30 miles away. She had taken two trains and a bus—a two-hour journey.

I then said to Iris, "This breast must mean a lot to you, as you have to go through a lot to finish six weeks of radiation. You obviously want to keep your breast." She practically yelled in response, "I don't want to keep my breast, my surgeon does!"

I sent her back for a mastectomy and the surgeon was not too happy.

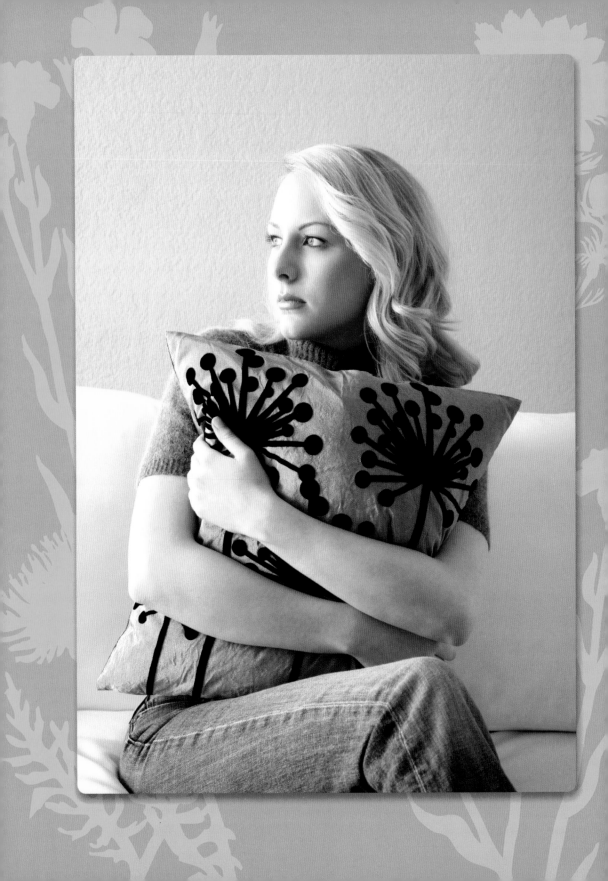

Control Point 3

What Will I Do about My Breast?

Control Point #3

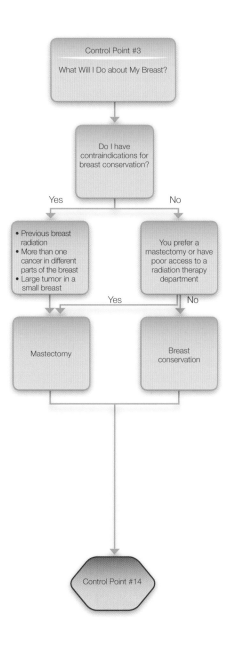

3

What Will I Do about My Breast?

A garden analogy

Two important decisions need to be made, and the first and most important decision is how your breast should be treated. The second is what to do about the lymph glands under your armpit (Figure 21).

Earlier, I mentioned that the breast can be compared to a rose bush in your garden and the cancer to a weed growing under it (Figure 22). The first and more "radical" option is to have the entire breast removed together with the cancer in it—known as a mastectomy. This is like a gardener removing the whole rose bush, getting out a large spade and leaving behind no evidence of the plant or the weed underneath (Figure 23). The less radical procedure is to remove the cancer with a healthy margin of normal breast tissue—known as breast conservation. This is like the gardener using a smaller spade and removing just the weed plus a small area of surrounding soil and keeping the rose bush (Figure 24).

The problem is that the weed can still come back even though the remaining soil looks clear. To reduce that risk, we need to smother any remaining seeds that may have been left behind when the weed was taken out. In a garden, we may use a weed mat, or some newspaper or straw mulch, but with breast cancer, we use a course of radiation therapy (Figure 25). Without radiation therapy, the risk of the cancer coming back can be as high as 30 percent over the next five to ten years following a lumpectomy and 5–10 percent if radiation is given.

PLEASE, PLEASE—do not rush this decision! Once the breast is gone, it cannot be put back!

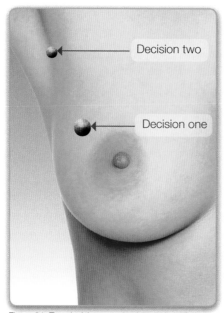

Decision two

Decision one

Figure 21: Two decisions need to be made at first: what to do about the breast, and what to do about the armpit.

There are two questions that you must answer at this point:

- Do I have the whole breast removed? Or . . .

- Do I have the lump removed with a lumpectomy and then have a course of radiation therapy lasting five to six weeks?

We know from Iris's story (page 65) that you may want a mastectomy; you may feel more comfortable with a mastectomy, but your surgeon may try to convince you to have a lumpectomy.

Before I go too much further, I'd like to point out that a clever doctor defined six different parts of the breast. These parts are the four "quadrants," the "central" part behind the nipple and **areola** (pigmented area around your nipple), and the "axillary tail," which is the part of the breast that extends toward your armpit (Figure 26). Knowing which quadrant or quadrants your cancer is in is important, particularly if your cancer involves more than one quadrant, when a mastectomy may be indicated; or is behind the nipple (central area), in which case the nipple may need to be removed if you want to keep your breast.

If you found a lump, the surgeon will feel the lump while you're under anesthetic and remove it with a rim of healthy tissue. If your cancer was only found on a mammogram or ultrasound and you and the surgeon cannot feel a lump, then a procedure called "wire localization" will be performed by a radiologist on the night before or the morning of your surgery. This involves inserting a guide wire (called a "hookwire") via X-ray or ultrasound control and positioning it just beyond your cancer. When you're under anesthetic, the surgeon will follow the wire to find and remove the cancer (where the tip of the wire, or the "hook," is), along with a rim of surrounding healthy tissue, and then remove the wire with the piece of breast tissue attached.

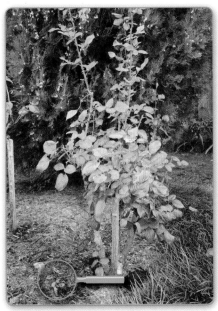

Figure 22: A weed under a rose bush—like a cancer in your breast.

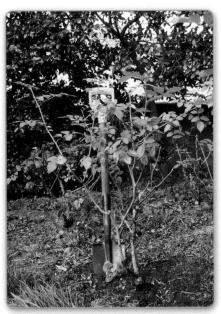

Figure 23: A mastectomy is like removing the weed and all of the rose bush with a large spade.

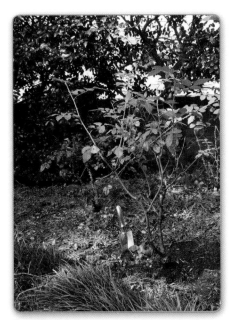

Figure 24: Breast conservation is like removing the weed with some of the normal-looking soil around it, while keeping the rose bush.

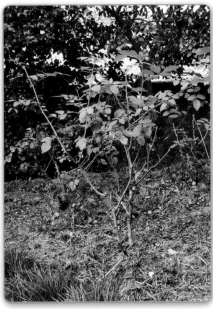

Figure 25: Giving a five- to six-week course of radiation is like putting straw mulch to starve any seeds that may have been left behind.

What Will I Do about My Breast?   71

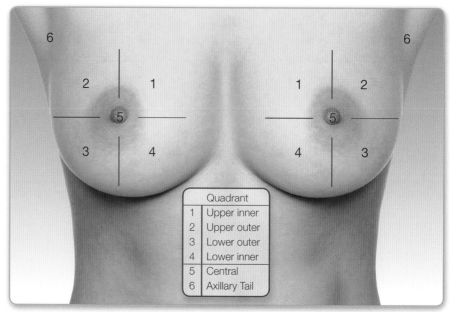

Quadrant	
1	Upper inner
2	Upper outer
3	Lower outer
4	Lower inner
5	Central
6	Axillary Tail

Figure 26: Different locations on the breast, called "quadrants."

Absolute indications for a mastectomy

The absolute *medical* reasons to have a mastectomy are:

- When there is more than one cancer in different quadrants of the breast. If there is a cancer, for example, at the 11 o'clock position, 50 mm (2 inches) above the nipple; and another at the 5 o'clock position, 80 mm (3 inches) below the nipple, then you are probably better off having a mastectomy. This situation is called **multicentric cancer** (Figure 27). On the other hand, if you have two or more cancers in the same quadrant that are quite close together and can still be removed with a clear margin, then there is absolutely no need to have a mastectomy. This situation is called **multifocal cancer** (Figure 28).

- If, as a child or a teenager, you had cancer that required radiation therapy. Some patients with a type of cancer of the lymph glands known as Hodgkin's lymphoma will have had radiation therapy in the past to the breast area that may make subsequent radiation therapy to the breast quite difficult.

- If you have a very large cancer particularly in a smaller breast

- If you just feel more comfortable having a mastectomy than going through five or six weeks of radiation

- If you are pregnant, you cannot receive radiation until you have delivered your baby, so a mastectomy may be more appropriate for you

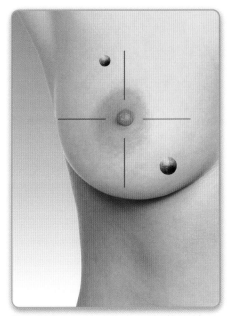 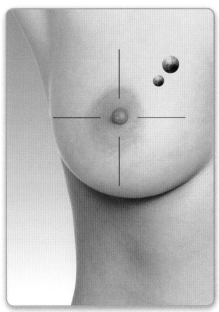

Figure 27: Two cancers in the breast (multicentric). One is at 11 o'clock and the other at 5 o'clock.

Figure 28: Two cancers close to each other (multifocal) at the 2 o'clock position of the right breast.

- Some pre-existing diseases (such as severe scleroderma or rheumatic diseases requiring high-dose steroids) may make you more prone to radiation complications, and a mastectomy may be less complicated

- If clear **margins** cannot be obtained after one or two breast conserving procedures.

Having a strong family history of breast cancer is not necessarily an indication for a mastectomy. Some doctors do occasionally recommend removing both breasts in this setting, but there is no consistent evidence that this increases your chance of surviving breast cancer (Recht 2009). Recht recently noted that some caregivers recommend a mastectomy for patients with strong family histories of breast cancer, or with a BRCA1 or 2 defect or mutation, because they feel that breast conservation is not effective in this group. He notes that this recommendation lowers the psychological barrier to removal of the normal breast. This has resulted, without strong research evidence, in removing both breasts for patients with strong family histories. However, he reports that most studies have found little or no difference in the chance of cancer coming back after breast conservation for patients with or without the breast cancer gene.

I remember advising Claire, who came to see me after having been recommended for a mastectomy by another multidisciplinary team. The problem was that the pathologist found a 2 mm area of DCIS next to an 11 mm area of invasive cancer as in Figure 27.

The pathologist called this multifocal, and the recommendation of that team was that the patient have a mastectomy.

When the patient came to see us, we did not know about the other opinion and we gave both options (mastectomy or breast conservation) as being *equally viable*. We advised her that a wide local excision (or lumpectomy) was perfectly adequate treatment. We reassured her that DCIS is often associated with cancer (as mentioned in Figure 6, it is usually the step before cancer) and that it is not uncommon to have one or more "satellite" lesions associated with the main tumor. Claire was very angry. She was not impressed that her team had recommended a mastectomy based on some *outdated theory* that if you have more than one tumor in the same quadrant, you need a mastectomy.

In fact, at the latest consensus conference (where a group of experts get together to establish guidelines), all panel members agreed that a mastectomy was not essential when there are two tumors in the same quadrant that can be excised in one operation (Schwartz 2006). The problem is that some surgeons do not read these guidelines, and therefore make decisions based on outdated science or snippets of information they learned through their general training.

The difference between a breast surgeon and a general surgeon

Surgeons are always trained first as general surgeons, and then they usually specialize in a field such as brain, heart, or breast surgery, particularly if they work in a large hospital or academic university hospital. If you can, consult a breast surgeon who sees and treats breast cancer every single day. Take care if your surgeon spends a lot of his or her week doing gallbladders, hemorrhoids, varicose veins, or colorectal cancer and only operates on the occasional patient with breast cancer.

Ask your surgeon, "Do you treat conditions other than breast cancer—just in case we needyou for something else?" It's a bit of a trick question, but this is a polite way of trying to work out if he or she is a general surgeon rather than a "breast surgeon." I do, however, exclude very experienced rural surgeons. It's impossible for every country town or small state to have a breast surgeon. My experience of these country surgeons is that they provide an exceptional service and work very hard to keep up to date and link in with experienced breast surgeons by telephone, email, or video conference.

Remember that an experienced general car mechanic in the country may still be better than the young Ford mechanic in the city. You can ask the surgeon, "What proportion of your work is breast disease?" Remember that very busy breast surgeons

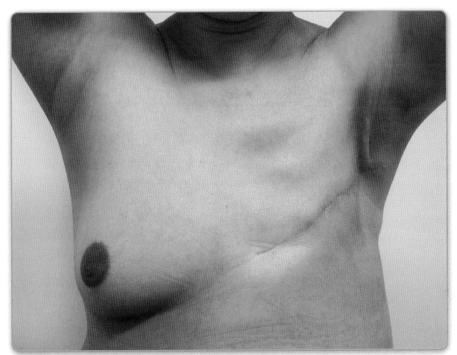

Figure 29: A mastectomy scar with dissolving "sub-cuticular" stitches under the skin.

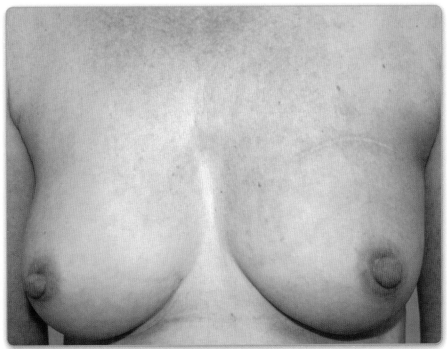

Figure 30: A good breast conservation scar with preservation of the shape, shown here four weeks after completing radiation and six months after surgery.

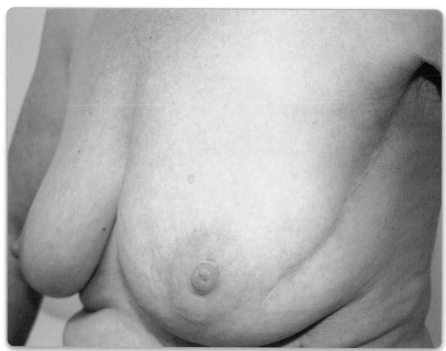

Figure 31: This patient has had a "quadrantectomy" to remove her breast cancer and a sentinel node biopsy done using the same incision extended into the armpit.

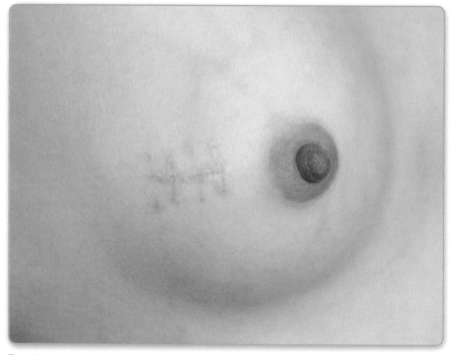

Figure 32: An example of a badly placed scar with obvious cross-hatching or "railroad tracks"

may focus 80–90 percent of their practice on breast disease and 10 percent on hormone conditions such as thyroid disease.

Some surgeons sub-specialize in cancer operations (surgical oncologist), and some may focus on both breast cancer and melanoma (a type of skin cancer). Breast surgeons know about **sentinel node mapping** and the **sentinel node biopsy** technique, explained in the next chapter, and generally work in a team that includes at least a radiation oncologist and a medical oncologist.

Some surgeons are now trained in advanced plastic surgery techniques to reshape the remaining breast after your cancer is removed. This is sometimes referred to as oncoplastic surgery. Your surgeon may also discuss adjusting the appearance of your other breast to more closely match your treated breast. This is often known as "contralateral symmetrization". **Skin-sparing mastectomy** is also gaining popularity where the breast tissue is removed through a small scar without removing all of the overlying skin. The breast mound is then recreated and the natural shape and contour of the breast is preserved, using either a permananent implant or tissue flap. In some patients, with very early disease, the nipple can be preserved (Patani, 2008).

Remember, a doctor's personality isn't everything. One of my patients insisted on seeing three different plastic surgeons. She went with the one with the best personality but wasn't happy with the final result Also important is their ability to do nice wounds with stitches under the skin, if possible. These are called sub-cuticular stitches (Figures 29–31), and are preferable to "railroad tracks," or cross-hatching, where the stitches are applied outside the skin at right angles to the main incision (Figure 32). Sub-cuticular stitches dissolve on their own and leave a less obvious scar than external stitches or staples, which need to be removed by your surgeon. When deciding on a surgeon, insist on seeing some pictures of their own work.

The chance of recurrence after breast conservation or a mastectomy is the same!

Assuming you have a choice between a mastectomy or breast conservation, I would like to reassure you that no one choice is better than the other. Some surgeons tell their patients that a mastectomy has a lower risk of cancer recurrence than breast conservation. Some patients then feel pressured to choose a mastectomy, as it appears on first look to be "better."

Based on the results of very large **clinical trials**, the overall recurrence rates are the same either way (Figure 33). So let's look at the risk of recurrence in the breast (after breast conservation) or chest wall ten years after a mastectomy. A recurrence in the chest wall looks like small pimples or reddish nodules, and a recurrence in the

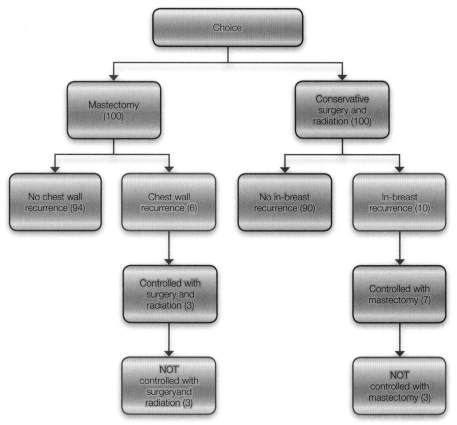

Figure 33: Mastectomy or breast conservation and the chance of a recurrence in the breast or chest wall ten years after treatment.

breast usually appears as a lump or an abnormality on a mammogram. The average risk of a chest-wall recurrence is about six in 100, or 6 percent. If this occurs, it can be brought back under control for 50 percent of such patients (that is, three of the six) by further surgery and radiation therapy. The ultimate risk of having an uncontrolled chest-wall recurrence if a mastectomy is chosen is three in 100, or 3 percent (the last red box on the left in Figure 33). The problem here is that all 100 women who chose a mastectomy have had to live with the trauma of losing their breast.

If breast conservation is chosen, then the chance of the cancer coming back in the breast within a ten-year period is ten in 100, or 10 percent. Seven of these ten women can have a mastectomy, but in three, the cancer comes back in such a way that it's inoperable. In this scenario, 90 have a conserved breast; seven have a mastectomy; and similar to the risk after a mastectomy, three have disease that is uncontrolled (the last red box on the right in Figure 33).

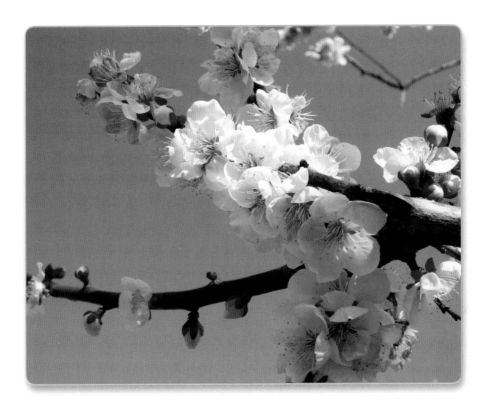

So basically, the ultimate chance of cancer coming back (after we include the chance of getting a recurrence back under control) is the same. Three patients will have a problem either way. Further, the long term results of large clinical trials have shown that treatment by mastectomy or conservative surgery and radiation give equivalent survival rates.

CONTROL POINT #3 – WHAT WILL I DO ABOUT MY BREAST?

WARNING Do not rush this decision! Once the breast is gone, it cannot be put back!

TIP Understand the difference between a breast surgeon and a general surgeon. Breast surgeons know about the sentinel node biopsy technique and generally work in a team with oncologists.

REMEMBER If you want a mastectomy and feel more comfortable with a mastectomy rather than radiation treatment, go with your gut feeling. Understand the risks and benefits of keeping or losing your breast.

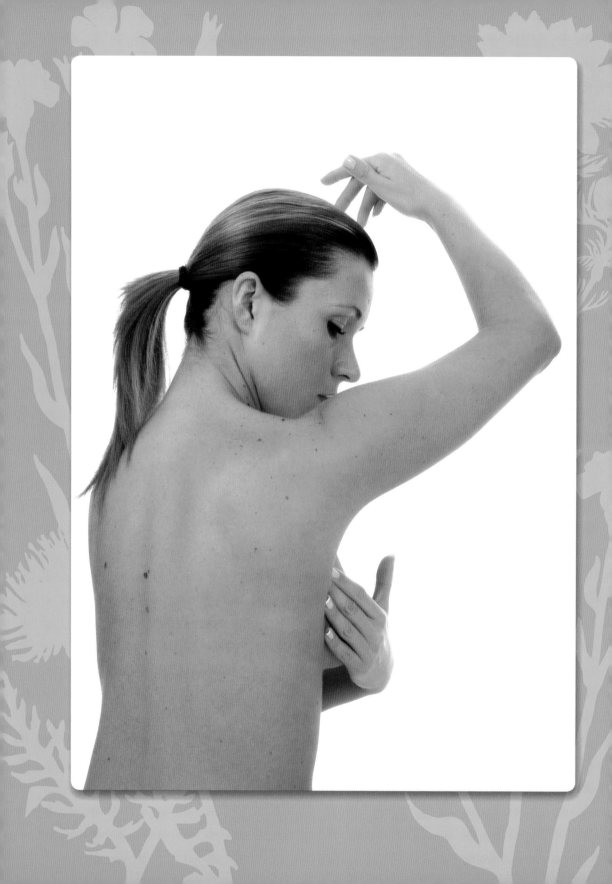

Control Point 4

What Will I Do about My Armpit?

Control Point #4

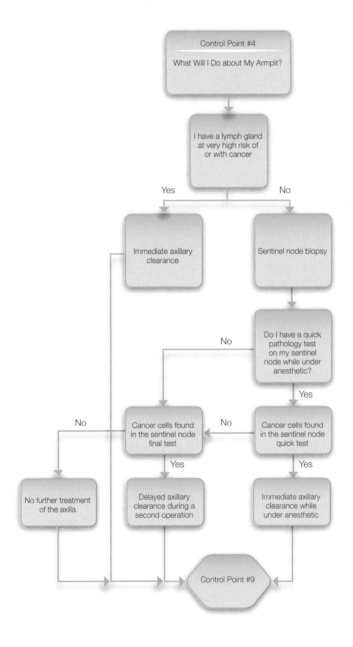

Control Point #4

What Will I Do about My Armpit?

I have a lymph gland at very high risk of or with cancer

Yes

No

Immediate axillary clearance

Sentinel node biopsy

Do I have a quick pathology test on my sentinel node while under anesthetic?

No

Yes

Cancer cells found in the sentinel node final test

No

Cancer cells found in the sentinel node quick test

No

Yes

Yes

No further treatment of the axilla

Delayed axillary clearance during a second operation

Immediate axillary clearance while under anesthetic

Control Point #9

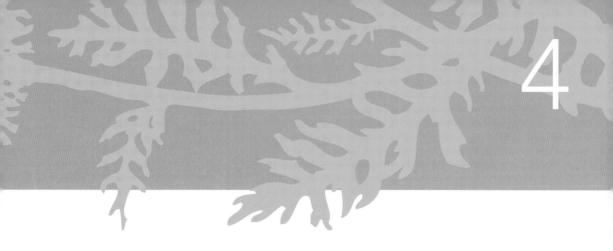

4

What Will I Do about My Armpit?

Understanding the lymphatic system surrounding your breast

The second important pre-operative decision is what to do about your armpit or axilla. You will recall that earlier, on page 33, I likened the way breast cancer can spread to the idea of a rosebush in a garden patch, with the lymph glands in your armpit being in the adjacent garden patch.

The axilla is a pad of fat that contains lots of lymph glands, or "**nodes.**" Lymph glands are located in many parts of the body and are part of the immune system, which helps us fight infections and cancer. For example, when you have a sore throat from the common cold, the lymph glands are often tender and enlarged because the infection is being attacked and stopped by the lymph glands. The same thing happens with breast cancer.

The lymph glands in the body are connected by the **lymphatic system**. The lymphatic system includes not only the lymph glands or "**lymph nodes,**" but also a network of tiny channels connecting all the glands called **lymph vessels**. The first draining lymph gland from the involved breast is called the **sentinel node**, and it receives multiple lymphatic channels from the area in the breast where your cancer started. The sentinel node is a type of "guardian" lymph gland, and it is thought that the lymphatic vessels drain there first before being connected by the lymph vessels to other lymph glands. There are usually one to three sentinel nodes draining each breast.

The lymph vessels carry fluid around the body, mainly under our skin, to lymph glands in the armpit, groin, neck, and elsewhere. The lymphatic system acts to fight infection, control the immune system, and help to get rid of some of the body's waste products. Antibodies to fight infection are made by the lymphatic system, and some waste products are broken down in the lymph glands.

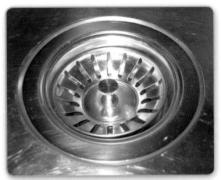

Figure 34: A lymph gland is a bit like a drain in your kitchen sink—it acts as a filter to stop cancer cells (in this case, a pea) from traveling any further.

Breast cancer can spread to the lymph glands via the lymphatic system, and they are often the first port of call. Our lymph glands and our immune system are trying to stop the cancer from spreading any further. In many ways, the lymph glands are like a filter trap in a sink (Figure 34).

Figure 35 shows how the lymph glands are organized in the armpit around the pectoralis minor muscle, which is the muscle under the pectoralis major muscle (not shown). It is the pectoralis major that most people call "the pec," and it is prominent in weightlifters. My research has shown that there is an average of 25 lymph glands in three separate areas, or "levels," of the armpit. There are about 15 lymph glands in level I, about seven lymph glands in level II, and about two to three lymph glands in level III. The highest point of the armpit is level III of the axilla, and it's about one inch (2.5 cm) from the **supra-sternal notch**. This is the notch just above your breastbone, or sternum. These lymph glands are also called the **infra-clavicular glands**. Just above the highest point of the axillary glands are the lymph glands at the base of the neck above the collarbone. This area is called the "**SCF**," or **supra-clavicular fossa**. There are also some lymph glands between the ribs and the breastbone known as the "**IMC**," or **internal mammary chain** (Figure 35).

Deciding between a sentinel node biopsy or an axillary clearance

As with breast conservation versus mastectomy, there are also two surgical choices for dealing with the lymph glands. Very occasionally, radiation is also given to the axilla on its own or following surgery.

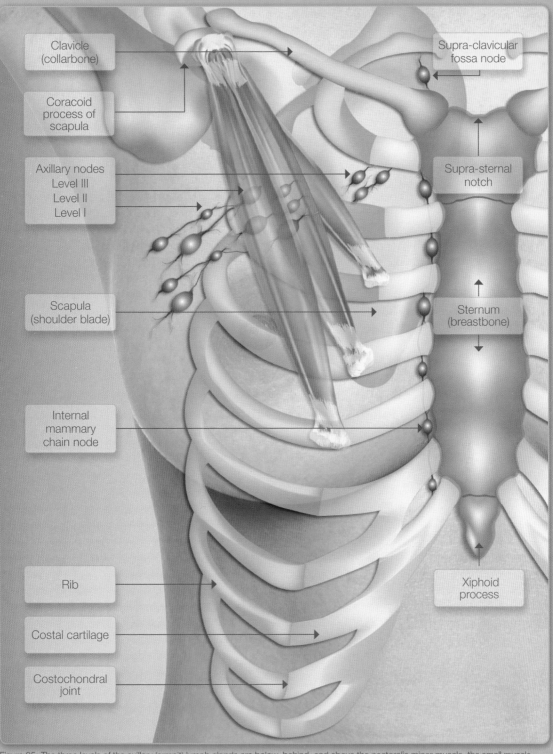

Clavicle
(collarbone)

Coracoid
process of
scapula

Axillary nodes
Level III
Level II
Level I

Scapula
(shoulder blade)

Internal
mammary
chain node

Rib

Costal cartilage

Costochondral
joint

Supra-clavicular
fossa node

Supra-sternal
notch

Sternum
(breastbone)

Xiphoid
process

Figure 35: The three levels of the axillary (armpit) lymph glands are below, behind, and above the pectoralis minor muscle, the small muscle behind the pectoralis major (not shown). Other lymph glands are located above the collarbone (supra-clavicular fossa) and beside the breastbone (internal mammary chain).

And again, it's very important not to rush this decision either. The options are:

1. A sentinel node biopsy, where only the first gland on the same side of the breast cancer is removed, and if that is clear, no further lymph glands are taken. Or …

2. An "**axillary clearance**," where some or all of the lymph glands from under the armpit are removed either during the mastectomy or breast conservation, or following a sentinel node biopsy that revealed cancer. Dissection or clearance involves removing the pad of fat in the armpit that contains the lymph glands, while being careful to protect the blood vessels and nerves (Figure 36). Many surgeons still also recommend a sentinel node biopsy even if they decide with you to perform an immediate axillary clearance, as it can give them extra guidance during the procedure.

This can be a difficult concept to grasp, so I will go back to my garden example. Having a sentinel node mapping procedure and biopsy is a bit like finding a "runner" from the weed under the rose bush and following it into the next garden patch, then using a small spade to dig around the runner to see if it's taken root there as well. If the runner hasn't taken root and there are no weeds in the next garden patch then removing some of the soil in that patch will not be necessary after examination with our small spade (sentinel node biopsy). If it has, then we will need a bigger spade to check all of the second patch and remove any weeds (axillary clearance).

When my son was a lot younger, he used to come home from school with homework and projects. This was always a very stressful time for me because I am not at all practical. I cannot make things and usually break things—this is why I'm not a surgeon. One year, my son came home with a science project on radiation. At last, something I knew a bit about! In fact, I learned something from his project. When plumbers want to know the location of underground pipes, they can pour some

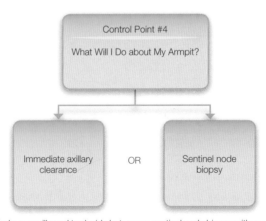

Figure 36: Pre-operatively, you will need to decide between a sentinel node biopsy with or without an axillary clearance.

radioactive fluid down the drain and use Geiger counters to find out where the pipes are and dig in the right spot. This is exactly what takes place in the sentinel node procedure: radioactive dye is injected around a breast cancer, and over the next hour or two, it drains into the first filter trap, or sentinel lymph node. The radioactive dye in the sentinel node shows up on an X-ray taken using a gamma camera. Just as the radioactivity that collects in the first downpipe is picked up by the plumber, who then knows where a pipe blockage may be located without having to excavate the whole room, the surgeon can carefully remove the sentinel node without clearing all of your axilla.

You and your doctor will need to know whether or not the cancer has spread from the first garden patch (stage 1) or to the second patch (stage 2), as this determines not only your prognosis, but also how much treatment will be required for the second garden patch as well as the rest of the garden, or the rest of your body. As I will talk about later, if a seed has blown in the wind from the first garden patch to the adjacent patch, there is a higher chance that it may have blown to other parts of the garden (in other words, other parts of your body).

If a seed is found in the adjacent patch, then we nearly always use some sort of weed killer on the rest of the garden just in case a seed we can't see has gone further afield. In practical terms, when the lymph glands are involved, we normally recommend extra treatments like hormonal treatment or chemotherapy for "seeds" that may have escaped to other parts of the garden or the rest of the body.

Don't be complacent about how you are treated; ask your team about their own particular philosophy about how they will treat your armpit. It's important that you get the best possible "local control"—that is, ensure that the disease is treated well enough that it doesn't come back in the breast, chest wall, or surrounding lymph glands. I cannot emphasize this enough. We know now that local control is vitally important and may increase your chance of survival by 5 to 10 percent.

Think carefully about your choices regarding your armpit. Sentinel node biopsy is a smaller operation, but a negative result may be a "**false negative**." In other words, cancer may be left behind, but this is more of a problem with larger cancers, as I will show in Table 1 below. On the other hand, if it the cancer has already spread to the sentinel node, then you may need a second operation to get rid of the cancer in the remaining lymph glands.

What is the chance that the cancer has spread to the lymph glands?

Before I discuss the reasons that may help you and your doctor decide between a small or a larger operation for your armpit or axilla, it's very important to understand your own risk of cancer spreading from the breast to the armpit.

Table 1 below shows the chance of having a cancerous lymph gland involved in the armpit, based on the size of the cancer in your breast, and its grade (Coombs and Boyages 2007). Basically, the bigger a cancer or the higher its grade, the higher the risk of cancer spreading to the armpit. A 10 mm tumor has about a 20 percent chance of lymph gland involvement, whereas a 30 mm tumor has a 50 percent chance of involvement. You can work out the probability of lymph gland involvement as I show below, but it is quite mathematical, and if you do not want this amount of detail you can skip it and move onto the next section.

The best approach is to look at the size of the tumor in millimeters (using the ultrasound), multiply this by 1.5, and then add 6. This is the formula from some of my research: (size in mm on ultrasound x 1.5) + 6

For example, if your ultrasound found that you had a 20 mm tumor, then the probability of your lymph glands being involved is:

20 x 1.5 = 30, plus 6 = 36 percent, or over a one in three chance.

Sometimes, it's not worth playing the odds in such a situation. You may just want to know what's going on in the axilla rather than possibly having two separate operations: one for the sentinel node and then possibly an axillary clearance if the sentinel node is found to contain cancer cells during the final pathology testing.

The probability of nodal involvement by cancer, and the theoretical probability of retrieval of a false negative sentinel node biopsy, are shown in Table 1 for a grade 2 tumor, using an average false negative rate of 5 percent. The rates are slightly higher for a grade 3 tumor and slightly lower for a grade 1 tumor. The sentinel node biopsy is not a perfect test, and sometimes the results are "clear" or "negative," but if a full dissection were done, we would find cancer left behind in another (non-sentinel) gland, and hence it's called "false negative." The main reason a sentinel node biopsy is done is to avoid the higher complication rates that come with a full axillary clearance, such as pins and needles over the inner upper aspect of your arm and swelling of the arm, called **lymphedema**.

If you have a sentinel node biopsy and it is reported as clear or negative by the pathologist, we have to keep a close eye on your armpit to pick up any recurrence there quickly and remove it with a full axillary clearance if one occurs. Nobody really knows yet whether clearing the axilla immediately is better than waiting to see if cancer comes back due to a false negative sentinel node biopsy that results in a delay of the required treatment. What we do know is that the chance of cancer coming back in the armpit is very low after a sentinel node biopsy.

In Table 1, if your tumor is like the first example (5 mm), then a sentinel node biopsy is a good idea because the likelihood of finding cancer in the axilla is 13.5 percent and the likelihood of cancer being missed by a sentinel node biopsy is less than 1

Tumor Size (mm)	Percent Risk of a Positive Sentinel Node	Percent Risk of a False Negative Sentinel Node
5	13.5%	0.7%
10	21.0%	1.1%
15	28.5%	1.4%
20	36.0%	1.8%
25	43.5%	2.2%
30	51.0%	2.6%
40	66.0%	3.3%
50	81.0%	4.1%

Table 1: Relationship between tumor size, the risk of cancer spreading to the armpit, and the chance that a sentinel node biopsy will miss cancer ("false negative")

percent. The estimated false negative rate is calculated by multiplying the "Percent Risk of a Positive Sentinel Node" by the average false negative rate of 5 percent. The last row of the table shows that if your tumor is about 50 mm wide (about 2 inches), then there is an 81 percent chance of your glands being involved ([50 x 1.5] + 6 = 81) and over a 4 percent chance (81 x 0.05 = 4.1) that if your test result is negative, it's a false negative. In this situation, it may not be worth taking the gamble of not having a full axillary clearance done. However, see what your surgeon and if necessary your oncologist thinks, and ultimately go with your own gut feeling after they have answered all your questions.

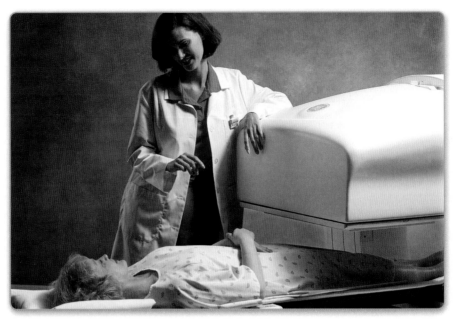

Figure 37: A gamma camera, which picks up the low-dose radiation emitted from your sentinel node.

How a sentinel node biopsy is done

For a sentinel node procedure to be successful, you need a good team of doctors who work well together. You need a radiologist to inject the radioactive dye and read the subsequent X-rays, and usually the surgeon will inject a blue dye around the cancer while you're anesthetised. That dye can be taken up by the lymphatics and drain to the sentinel node. You also need a surgeon who has the right equipment, including a probe like a Geiger counter that can detect the radiation in the sentinel node. The sentinel node is found, or "mapped," using up to three techniques. These are:

- A nuclear medicine test called **lymphoscintigraphy** (lymphatic mapping) that's performed before the operation

- A scan using a handheld probe performed by the surgeon during surgery

- A blue dye test, also performed by the surgeon as part of the operation

Lymphoscintigraphy (lymphatic mapping)

Typically, a tiny amount of a radiation-labeled material called a colloid is injected above or around the tumor, or sometimes around the nipple. The radioactive materials, trapped by the draining sentinel lymph nodes, are seen with a special X-ray machine called a gamma camera (Figure 37) as "hot spots" one or two hours after the injection of the colloid (Figure 38). The big advantage of this technique is that it allows sentinel

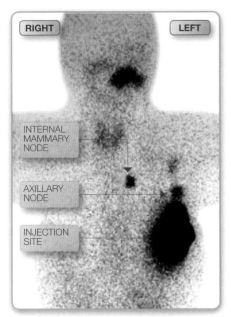

Figure 38: A sentinel node scan done before surgery, showing uptake behind the breastbone, in the armpit, and around the breast tumor.

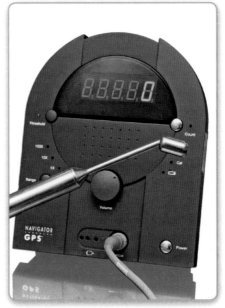

Figure 39: A type of Geiger counter used to detect the "hot" sentinel nodes during surgery.

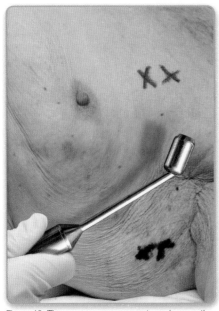

Figure 40: The surgeon uses a scan to probe over the marks put on your skin over the sentinel node.

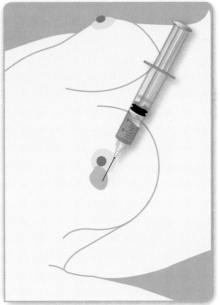

Figure 41: Blue dye is injected as the first part of the surgical procedure just after you are anesthetised.

lymph nodes not found in the armpit (such as those next to the breastbone, called internal mammary chain nodes) to be seen. The locations of these nodes are then often marked on the skin with a waterproof marker to help the surgeon know where to make their cut and start looking for the gland (see "X" marks in figure 40).

Don't be frightened about this test. It uses very low-dose radiation. Your doctors will usually use a local anesthetic before injecting the dye (and maybe you should insist on it). And remember that just because your sentinel nodes are being mapped, this doesn't mean that the cancer has spread to them.

This test shows the first downpipe and helps your plumber (in this case, your surgeon) to know exactly where to dig—to find the spot where it's most likely for the cancer to spread first. In the example shown, the lymphatics have taken up the dye in two directions to the lymph glands behind the breastbone (IMC or internal mammary chain) and the axilla.

Handheld probe

This is the Geiger counter (Figure 39) used to find the sentinel nodes that the nuclear physician has marked on the skin and that are shown in the X-ray above. Usually, the surgeon double checks the area, because sometimes sentinel nodes are "hot" (radioactive), as shown by the probe (Figure 40), but were not visible on the X-ray, usually because of technical reasons.

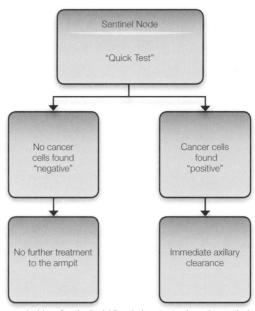

Figure 42: What the surgeon decides after the "quick" pathology test, where the sentinel node is tested while under anesthetic.

Blue dye

Intra-operative blue dye is injected during the operation and taken up by lymphatic channels and nodes, allowing your surgeon a second way to see the sentinel node (the first is the Geiger counter probe). Figure 41 shows how blue dye is injected as the first part of the surgical procedure just after you are put under the anesthetic. Don't worry, you won't feel the needle at all.

A combination technique is ideal but don't worry too much if they use one technique over another. It really depends on the expertise and the resources the surgeon possesses.

A "quick test" can be done on the removed sentinel node while you are under anesthetic

Cancer that has spread to the sentinel node is sometimes found during the operation, while you are still asleep. There are two ways of doing this:

- The sentinel node that has been removed is sent urgently to the pathologist, who cuts it in half and swipes it across a slide, a bit like a Pap smear slide. This is then quickly examined to look for cancer cells.

- A second approach is called a **frozen section**, where the sentinel node is frozen and then quickly stained and examined. Another more recent variation involves a pathology technician placing a few slices of the sentinel node in a specially designed machine that runs a range of tests on the gland, looking for special staining or genetic changes and confirming if a cancer cell is found in the sentinel node (Mansel 2009).

The reason for the quick test is that the surgeon can immediately talk to the pathologist and ask if any cancer cells can be seen in the sentinel node. The pathologist is under a lot of pressure at this point, because only a small slice of the sentinel node is looked at very quickly while you're still asleep.

The advantage of this quick test is that it *may prevent you from needing two anesthetics and two operations*. In other words, if the sentinel node is positive, it's better to know immediately so they can remove the remaining lymph glands and do an axillary clearance right then and there. But a word of caution: not all hospitals around the world have a pathologist on standby to do these quick tests, and it's still better to study the sentinel node carefully after you leave hospital than it is to have an immediate axillary clearance. Figure 42 shows the possible outcome after a quick test.

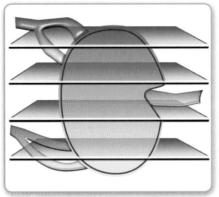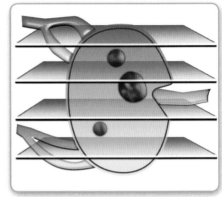

Figure 43: The sentinel node is sliced about six times in search of any cancer cells (shown on the right in red). The gland on the left is negative.

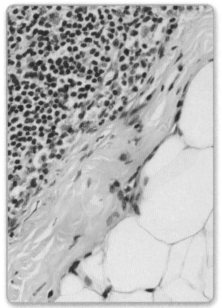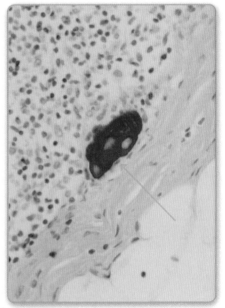

Figure 44: A sentinel node as seen with the naked eye (left), and with special immuno-histochemical (IHC) stain. The red spot on the right is called a micro-metastasis (arrowed).

Slower, more accurate testing of the sentinel node the week after your surgery

The problem with these quick tests on the sentinel node is that they're only about 70 percent accurate. The only way to really study the sentinel node is to cut it up into about six pieces and examine lots of sections during the week after your surgery (Figure 43). In addition, the naked eye does not see all of these small cells, which are often smaller than a grain of sand. We need to use a special stain called an **immuno-histochemistry (or IHC) stain**, which can sometimes show the cancer cells as black, dark brown or red.

Figure 44 is an example of a sentinel node as seen by a pathologist under a microscope. The purple section is unstained by immuno-histochemistry and shows no visible cancer cells, but on the right side, with the IHC stain added, there are some red cells visible—these are cancer cells.

There is a lot of controversy about what small deposits of cancer cells in a sentinel node really mean when found by the more sensitive IHC method. I'm a member of the international committee for the staging system for breast cancer, which looks at how breast cancer should be classified. In 2007, I was sent over 20 articles that had been published in medical journals that looked at how small deposits called **micrometastases** or micromets, or even smaller deposits called **isolated tumor cells** or "**ITCs**," impact on a patient's prognosis.

The international classification committee has tried to differentiate "minor" spread to the armpit, or isolated tumor cells (ITCs), from micrometastases primarily on the basis of size. ITCs are defined as single cells or small clusters of cells not greater than 0.2 mm in largest dimension and are classified as pN0(i). Micro-metastases are defined as tumor deposits greater than 0.2 mm, but not greater than 2.0 mm in largest dimension. Cases in which only micrometastases are detected (i.e., not greater than 2 mm) are classified pN1mi. Where cancer is greater than 2 mm, this is called a **macro-metastasis**.

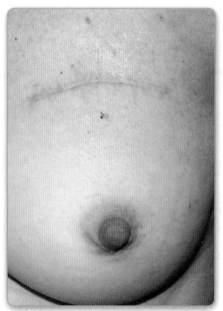

Figure 45: Blue stain on the skin after a Patent Blue injection may take several days or weeks to resolve and may be confused with a bruise.

After reading all the latest publications, my view was not to worry too much if all you have is ITCs. These ITCs in the sentinel node may simply be "visitors" and harmless, rather than "residents," which can lodge and start growing. Just because a cell is dislodged doesn't mean it's dangerous. In the sink example above, just because a pea falls into the sink and gets caught, that doesn't mean it's going to grow there (Figure 34). Patients with micro-metastases tend to do better than those with macro-metastases, but they still have a small impact on reducing survival and therefore should be taken into account when deciding about chemotherapy or hormonal treatment.

The blue dye may turn your urine blue-green for about 24 hours. The blue dye is sometimes confused with a bruise, which can also occur after surgery. The skin over your breast may be stained blue for three to four weeks, but this is rarely permanent (Figure 45). Mild allergic reactions can occur in 1 to 2 percent of patients. Severe allergic reactions are extremely rare. If this occurs, it usually causes no serious problem, because your anesthetist is watching closely over you.

I was teaching some technicians at one stage and asked one of the young men who was helping me plan a patient's radiotherapy what could have caused the blue mark on the breast. Without blinking an eyelid he said, "Was it because you examined the patient too hard and bruised her?" He will never forget that lesson and we still have a laugh about it from time to time.

Lymphedema is swelling of the arm that occurs after axillary treatment of any sort (dissection, radiation, or even after a sentinel node biopsy). The risk is estimated to be 1 to 2 percent after a sentinel node biopsy. However, the results of the studies to date show that a sentinel node biopsy is safe for the majority of women because:

- It's a far smaller procedure with fewer immediate complications than an axillary clearance

- There is less chance of long-term shoulder or arm problems compared to a full axillary clearance

- If your cancer is small, there is a high chance that your lymph glands will be not be involved with cancer and an axillary clearance is therefore an unnecessary procedure

- It allows mapping of lymph gland areas that a surgeon may not normally dissect, such as the level II or III axillary nodal region or internal mammary chain

- The risk involved in leaving a trace of cancer behind (a false negative) is very low, particularly if you are having other treatments such as radiation therapy, chemotherapy, or hormonal treatment

- The risk of leaving cancer cells behind is higher for cancers over 50 mm or when there is more than one cancer in the breast (multifocal or multicentric tumors). Clinical trials are underway looking at the safety of sentinel node biopsy in this setting

- The biological significance of small traces of cancer, called isolated tumor cells or ITCs, is unclear, but they are very unlikely to influence your prognosis

- Very importantly, surgeons who practice sentinel node procedures usually have a specific interest and expertise in breast cancer and tend not to be general surgeons.

My overall view is that it is a safe first procedure to see whether the first node is involved, and a final decision about whether to proceed to an axillary clearance can then be taken based on the result.

How an axillary clearance is done

The second option for the axilla, instead of or in addition to a sentinel node biopsy, is an **axillary clearance** or dissection, where some or all of the lymph glands are taken out of the armpit. This is the "gold standard" for assessing the extent of any disease in lymph glands in the axilla. For some patients, an axillary clearance is the best approach. For example, if you already have proven disease in your armpit, your surgeon will most likely recommend an axillary dissection with or without a sentinel node biopsy. Many surgeons will still do a sentinel node mapping procedure, even if they plan to do an axillary clearance, to help guide their dissection. An axillary clearance is also done immediately if your sentinel node is found to be involved with cancer, either via your "quick test" or when the final test is available.

An axillary clearance is a more complex and longer operation than the sentinel node biopsy, as the surgeon must carefully dissect the fat containing your lymph glands from around nerves, blood vessels, and muscles (Figure 35). It involves having a drain (a plastic tube) left in your armpit for about seven to ten days. The drain will remove fluid from under the skin that otherwise would build up due to incisions in the tissue that cause the small lymphatics and blood vessels under your skin to leak. This fluid is called **serous fluid** and is the same straw-colored serous fluid that can accumulate in a blister after sunburn.

Typically, once the drainage is down to fewer than 30 to 40 mL a day, the drain tube can be pulled out. Sometimes after the drain has been removed, you will continue to accumulate fluid around your scar. You will know when this is happening as you will experience some difficulty in getting your arm down against your side because of swelling. This is called a "**seroma**." This seroma fluid will need to be aspirated or drained by a radiologist, the surgeon, or a breast care nurse. Seromas are different from **hematomas**, which contain blood like a bruise, and from an **abscess**, which contains pus from an infection.

Absolute reasons to have an axillary clearance

The absolute reasons to have an axillary clearance include when:

- You have a gland in the armpit that feels like cancer, or preferably a **fine needle aspiration biopsy** or **core biopsy**—that showed cancer cells
- You have a large cancer and you're not prepared to take a chance that the sentinel node is going to be clear (see Table 1)
- The sentinel node quick test is positive
- The sentinel node final test is positive
- There is a lump in the armpit that is cancer, but the mammogram is clear (this is called **occult breast cancer**). This is a special situation that is a little complicated to treat, and opinions vary as to whether a mastectomy should be done or not.

Why is an axillary clearance important?

An axillary clearance is important because:

- It allows us to understand how many lymph glands are involved in the armpit and work out your prognosis
- If the lymph glands are involved, a clearance is good treatment and the chances of cancer coming back in the armpit are very low
- It allows radiation therapy to be restricted to the breast, which is less complicated and has fewer side effects than treating the gland areas as well
- Knowing the number of lymph glands involved helps us to decide whether you need hormonal treatment, chemotherapy, or both
- Some studies have suggested that a good axillary clearance may be associated with a better cure rate if your lymph glands are involved with cancer.

How many lymph glands should be removed from the armpit?

There is some variation in the extent of an **axillary dissection** or clearance of the lymph glands from the armpit. Most surgeons around the world clear most of the level I nodes and some or all of level II nodes. A few surgeons clear right up to level III. Some surgeons simply do a "sample," where only a few lymph glands in the first level are taken. Nobody really knows if it's important to take out all the lymph glands, particularly because it's thought that more surgery in the armpit may mean a greater chance of arm swelling, or lymphedema.

Most breast cancer experts prefer to clear the axilla sufficiently that at least 15 lymph glands are found by the pathologist. However, many factors influence the number of lymph glands found under your armpit following an axillary clearance. For example, there are fewer lymph glands when you've had chemotherapy before your surgery.

The good news is that the famous American surgeon, Bernard Fisher (to whom we are all eternally grateful for his innovative research over the last 40 years or so), has really helped our understanding of recurrence rates and treatment of the armpit.

The pathologist may record the number of involved nodes in your pathology report as "0/5" or "0/17," meaning that your breast cancer had not spread to any of five or seventeen nodes that were found. If cancer has not spread to the lymph glands, then this is often called "node negative"; and if it has spread, it is called "node positive."

Finding "4/7" means that four lymph glands contained cancer out of seven found, and the concern here is that any lymph glands left behind may contain cancer and need more treatment, such as radiation therapy. We would have more confidence or certainty of what is really going on in the armpit if the count was "4/20," for example. Think of it as having a small brown paper bag full of red and black jellybeans.

If you really don't like black ones, and you grab a handful from the bag and find you have four blacks and three reds ("4/7"), then you may be worried that there are still a lot of black ones left behind because the mix appears to be roughly half and half.

That's like the pathologist finding four lymph glands involved with cancer and three not involved, which would leave him or her unsure of what's left in the remainder of the armpit.

But if you take two handfuls from the paper bag and find four black and 16 red jellybeans (that is, "4/20" are black), then you can be more confident about the real color mix in the bag.

A Danish study found that the surgeon and the pathologist have to find at least ten lymph glands in the armpit to be really confident about what's going on—to feel sure that they understand the "mix of red and black jellybeans" in your armpit (Axelsson 2009).

There is no doubt that the armpit portion of the operation is the most difficult, as this is the part that feels most uncomfortable. It does involve cutting a nerve that supplies some superficial skin in your upper arm, and surgeons often talk about this nerve having to be "sacrificed." Cutting this nerve causes some pins and needles in the upper and inner part of your arm, which can feel a bit strange. These pins and needles or intermittent sharp and sometimes shooting pains are worst in the first year or so. Whatever sensation or altered sensation is left after three years is generally how it will be in the long term.

Other side effects from an axillary clearance include the collection of fluid under the armpit (called a seroma) or, rarely, an infection. A good brochure, from the Westmead Breast Cancer Institute, on possible side effects and what needs to be done if they occur can be found at:

www.bci.org.au/images/stories/about_bc/factsheets/new_pdf/wound_care.pdf

A few years ago, I was involved in some research where, for several years, we followed a large group of women who had had breast surgery and axillary treatment and asked them all sorts of questions about this and other things related to their treatment. We found that the first three months is the worst time for discomfort in the arm, but the situation improves between months four and 12. How it feels at 12 months is how it will feel for the rest of your life (King 2000). This discomfort, although annoying, is not a serious complication, and hopefully it will slowly improve.

It's important to move your arm as quickly as possible after your drain is removed. One clinical trial compared patients who received early physical therapy (physiotherapy) to those who had received late physiotherapy, and it showed that patients who received early physiotherapy had better shoulder function in the long run (Bendz 2002). There should not be any activity that you did prior to surgery that you cannot resume after the initial recovery process. It's important to listen to your body and become attuned to your arm symptoms and general function. If you have had an axillary clearance, then you should regain your full range of motion within ten to 12 weeks after surgery. You should regain full range of motion within two to four weeks after a sentinel node biopsy without an axillary clearance. The only exception is if you have an immediate breast implant; in that case, it is best to avoid heavy household activities for the first six weeks after your surgery, but still use your full range of arm and shoulder motion and do some stretching exercises.

A good brochure on shoulder care, which includes these stretching exercises (including your fingers "climbing the wall", is found at:

www.bci.org.au/images/stories/about_bc/factsheets/new_pdf/shoulder_care.pdf

Remember that shoulder dysfunction can occur in the long term after treatment. Keep your shoulder active. See a physical therapist or physiotherapist as required. Remember, too, that radiation can sometimes cause some scarring or **fibrosis** in the pectoral muscle. This can be tender, but massaging the area with some moisturizer may help this, and may also help mobilize the arm. Get your partner or caregiver to help you with this.

In my experience, people whose posture is poor, or who sleep on their front or side and really twist their necks, can also suffer problems such as neck tenderness, headaches, pain radiating down the arm with pins and needles in the little finger of the affected side, and pain between their backbone and shoulder blade.

When this occurs, remember that it is not cancer, but rather usually related to your posture, or to the fact that you've changed the position in which you sleep after your surgery. It is very common. See a good physical therapist to help you get through this, and think about a physio pillow, which supports your neck a lot better while you sleep. There are some good neck exercises around. I like the ones at WebMD (with permission):

www.webmd.com/hw/health_guide_atoz/sig54597.asp

How to reduce your chances of lymphedema

Lymphedema of the arm is an accumulation of lymph fluid in the tissues of your arm, which causes swelling. Lymphedema can develop at any time after treatment for breast cancer. It usually starts in the first few years after treatment, but it is possible for it to start more than ten or even 20 years later. If you develop lymphedema, this does not mean that your breast cancer is coming back. Having surgery under your armpit increases the risk of scarring and what we call back-pressure. It's a bit like the difference between a fast flowing river, and a slow flowing river that is blocked by rocks. The one blocked by rocks backs up and the water is often murkier than a fast flowing river. Edema can also occur in your breast if it has been conserved, and this is discussed further in Chapter 14.

Early symptoms of lymphedema include heaviness, aching, and/or fluctuating swelling in the hands or fingers, or tightening of your rings. Later symptoms include swelling of the forearm or upper arm or the whole arm. These symptoms may initially settle overnight, but when more advanced, they can become permanent.

The more treatment you have to your armpit, the greater the risk of lymphedema. The risk of moderate or severe lymphedema (defined as more than a 20 mm difference in girth between your treated and untreated arm) is about 1.5 percent after a sentinel node biopsy, 7 percent after radiation, 8 percent after surgery, and 35 percent after

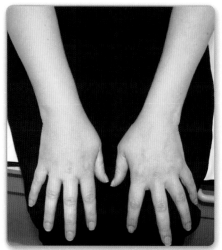

Figure 46: Moderate lymphedema or swelling in the fingers and back of the right hand and wrist area.

surgery together with radiation. Having chemotherapy, particularly taxanes, also increases the risk slightly.

If lymphedema does occur, it's usually mild and not very noticeable. But if it's moderate or severe and starts affecting your function, then treatments such as wearing a professionally fitted elastic compression sleeve or bandages, exercises, massage, and skin care may help. Figure 46 shows an example of someone who developed moderate lymphedema after surgery and radiation to the armpit. It can be difficult to tell the difference between the two sides but notice how the right wrist is slightly wider and there is some puffiness at the back of the hand.

The situation can become worse if there is as sudden increase in "traffic" — when the blood flow to your treated arm increases because of an infection, a burn, or overuse of the arm muscles because of excessive exercise. There have been a few cases of lymphedema occurring or increasing after a long flight.

If a river is blocked because of rocks, particularly if there is extra water from the rain, the river will breach its bank and flood the outside fields. The same thing can happen to your arm when there is a precipitating event like an infection. The fluid increases in volume and then seeps out into the soft tissues of your arm.

A particularly serious complication is **cellulitis**, where the fluid becomes infected and you may end up getting high temperatures and chills. This requires urgent antibiotics. If you have any sign of an infection, see your doctor to start antibiotics immediately.

Eighty percent of lymphedema cases develop in the first 12 months after surgery. Recent evidence has found that early detection and intervention may be the key to reducing the long-term development of irreversible "chronic" lymphedema. Technologies such as **bioimpedance** can detect early changes of fluid at a cellular level up to ten months earlier than detection with a tape measure. It's a good idea to be monitored at three- to six-monthly intervals in the first year after surgery to detect early signs before symptoms set in.

The good news is that more and more new treatments are being tried as more research into lymphedema is done. An occupational or physical therapist can explain your treatment options and help you to decide which is best for you. It takes a lot of patience and a bit of trial and error, so it's good to develop a partnership with your therapist. Taking control means feeling empowered to manage your own symptoms according to your lifestyle.

Exercise and movement are strongly recommended because muscle contraction helps to push the lymph fluid through the lymphatic channels, reducing the chance of swelling. Resuming an exercise program at the gym is encouraged too, as is participating in an "Encore" program, a free ten-week exercise program coordinated and funded by the YWCA in which women can participate at any stage of their breast cancer journey in a non-medical environment. Exercises are completed in a gym environment as well as in a heated pool.

See www.ywca.org (and search for "breast cancer") in the US or www.ywcaencore.org.au/ in Australia for more information.

Some good information is available at the Westmead Breast Cancer Institute at:

www.bci.org.au/images/stories/about_bc/factsheets/new_pdf/lymphoedema.pdf

and the National Cancer Institute at:

www.cancer.gov/cancertopics/pdq/supportivecare/lymphedema/

A really simple but important step in preventing infection after lymphedema is to keep your arm moisturized with a moisturizer that does not contain perfume, as perfume can irritate the skin. Massaging the arm daily in an upward direction assists the fluid in moving upward rather than staying in the arm. The lymphatics do not have a pump or one-way valves like your arteries, so rely on gentle massage and exercise to assist the movement and drainage of lymph fluid. Here are some other points:

Avoid repetitive movements:

- Do not overwork the affected arm

- Avoid repetitive movements such as excessive weightlifting, and if you're vacuuming, walk with the vacuum cleaner in a forward direction rather than moving your arm back and forth.

Movement is important, though, so the best approach is to resume your normal activities. If this involves, for example, lifting a 30-pound child several times a day, that's okay. Resume the activity gradually, though, and rest if you feel any heaviness, aching, or swelling in your arm. We know, for example, that Dragon Boat racing (Appendix 1) is a pretty intense type of exercise that does not induce lymphedema or make established lymphedema worse. More exercise and general activity increases the lymphatic pumping action, which is what we want, and it also makes you feel better psychologically.

Avoid cutting or damaging your skin:

- Use an electric razor for shaving, rather than a blade that could cut you and introduce infection

- Wear long gardening gloves when you do yard work

- Take care with sewing or quilting and use a thimble

- Take care of your fingernails and do not cut your cuticles

- Clean cuts with soap and water, and then use antibacterial ointment or an iodine preparation

- Avoid having blood tests or injections in the arm on the side of your surgery

- Avoid insect bites by using insect repellents.

Avoid constricting or restricting your arm

- Wear loose jewelry and wear clothes that do not constrict with tight bands or elastic

- Carry a handbag or shopping bag on the unaffected arm

- Do not use blood pressure cuffs on the affected arm

- When flying long distances, rest your arm in an elevated position and exercise it regularly during the flight. Ask for a window seat on the side of your affected arm so you have a ledge to prop your arm on, and consider wearing a compression sleeve.

- When sitting for long periods of time, such as during a long car or train journey, get up and have regular breaks to move around and stretch your muscles.

Avoid extreme temperatures

- Avoid extreme hot or cold, such as ice packs or heating pads and hot baths

- Avoid burns and use mitts when you are carrying hot food

- Try and avoid becoming too hot. Rest to cool down or go into an air conditioned environment

- Suntan gradually to avoid sunburn and skin peeling and always use sunscreen.

Despite this long list of dos and don'ts, the bottom line is to learn to listen to your body and don't go wrapping yourself in cotton wool.

CONTROL POINT #4 – WHAT WILL I DO ABOUT MY ARMPIT?

 WARNING Surgeons who don't practice sentinel node procedures tend to be general surgeons rather than specialized breast cancer surgeons

 TIP Moisturize your arm regularly after surgery, all the way up to your armpit, regardless of whether you've had a sentinel node biopsy or a full axillary clearance. Take extra care with your treated arm to minimize the chance of lymphedema.

 REMEMBER Talk to your surgeon about the advantages and disadvantages of a sentinel node biopsy versus a full axillary clearance. Don't rush this decision.

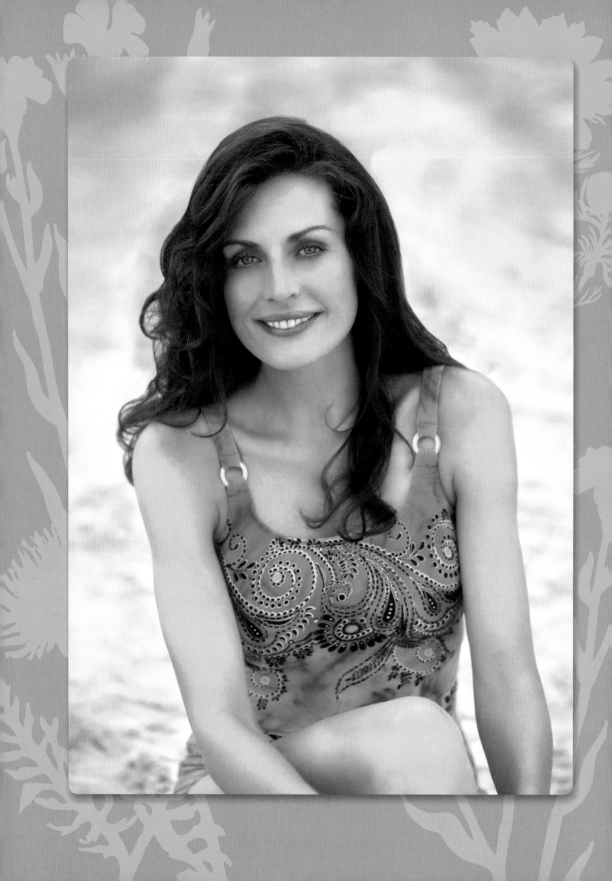

Control Point 5

If I Have a Mastectomy,
Can I Wear an External
Prosthesis?

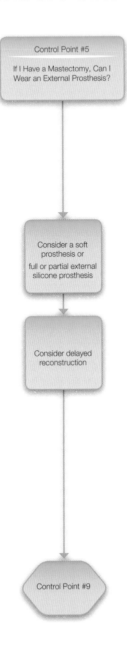

Control Point #5

If I Have a Mastectomy, Can I Wear an External Prosthesis?

Consider a soft prosthesis or
full or partial external silicone prosthesis

Consider delayed reconstruction

Control Point #9

5

If I Have a Mastectomy, Can I Wear an External Prosthesis?

If you don't have a reconstruction, getting a breast prosthesis is a good idea. This can be challenging at times and depends on how much support and information you get after your operation. The best people to talk to about a prosthesis are your discharge planner, social worker, or breast care nurse.Wearing an external prosthesis may help with your balance, symmetry, self-esteem and confidence.

What is a breast prosthesis?

A **breast prosthesis** is essentially an external, artificial breast shape or mound worn inside your bra or swimsuit. It's sometimes referred to as an external breast form. It is not an internal breast prosthesis or **implant**. Many women feel quite self-conscious after a mastectomy, because they may appear lopsided in clothes. A prosthesis can be temporary (usually lightweight) or permanent (weighted or lightweight) and some are suitable for active sports including swimming. All breast prostheses come in various skin tones and may be made from silcone or lighter materials.

What types of breast prostheses are available?

Ruth Handler (1916–2002) was an American businesswoman and president of the toy manufacturer Mattel, Inc., who is remembered primarily for her role in creating and marketing the BARBIE® doll (Figure 47). In the '70s, after having a mastectomy, she was not impressed with the quality of prostheses and started a company that produced the original NEARLY ME® line of breast prostheses. You'll probably want to buy two types of breast prostheses: a non-weighted and a weighted one.

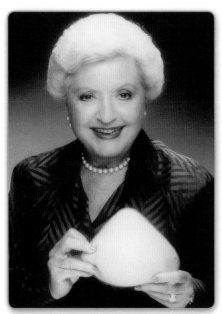

Figure 47: Ruth Handler, inventor of BARBIE® Doll and founder and creator of the original NEARLY ME® line of Breast Prostheses.

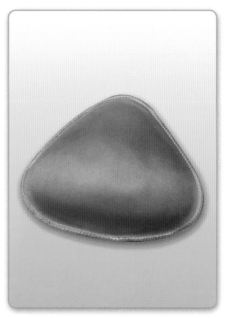

Figure 48: A soft-form or lightweight prosthesis.

A non-weighted foam or polyfill form is recommended when you're first recovering from surgery because it's softer and most comfortable over your healing skin (Figure 48). At the Institute where I work, we give these out for free. They're made by a local Zonta Club (www.Zonta.org), a part of Zonta International whose aim is to advance the status of women. Soft prostheses are also useful for informal leisure activities and feel good during warm weather and while swimming. They're conveniently machine-washable and lightweight. In different countries they may be called "comfies", "softies," "falsies" or a "filler." You may find that the soft-form prosthesis can "ride up" because it's so light. It may look better if you adjust the stuffing and pin it to the bottom of your bra cup. If you want to wear a bra with your soft prosthesis, try one that is soft and stretchy, without an underwire. Remember, your first bra after a mastectomy has to be easy to take on and off because your shoulder may be stiff at first if you have had surgery on your lymph glands.

Weighted silicone prostheses are still very soft but add the weight and balance that you need to reduce the potential for neck and back problems. They are hand-washable and look and feel better than soft prostheses because they're fitted to match the size, weight, and shape of your own breast. These too are worn externally and are not the same as breast implants. The added weight of a silicone prosthesis usually allows it to sit more easily at the same level as your other breast. If a silicone prosthesis "rides up," it might not be heavy enough.

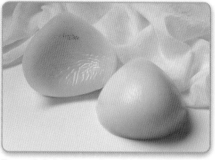 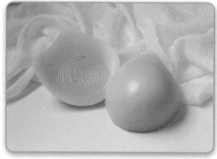

Figure 49: Soft silicone gel prostheses—(left) triangle (symmetrical), and (right) classical (asymmetrical).

After breast surgery, and also after radiation therapy, your chest area can be extra sensitive, so it's best to delay getting a silicone prosthesis until your chest area is fully healed after surgery, which generally takes about eight weeks. If you are having radiation treatment to the chest wall, wait at least six to eight weeks after it's completed and any skin reaction has settled.

You might want to ask your fitting service for a reassessment if you're not happy with how your prosthesis fits you. You really need to talk to your team about the style of your prosthesis , but the options include:

- Asymmetrical prostheses, often called classic style. One designed only for the left side and one only for the right side extend into the armpit (Figure 49, right).

- Symmetrical prostheses include the "pear shape" (also known as teardrop or oval prosthesis or the "triangle shape". The pear shape prostheses work on either side and can be worn sideways filling the area towards your arm, or straight up for center fullness and cleavage. Triangles, which are very popular, have been on the market since the early to mid-1990s and come in a large variety of shapes, skin tones, and weights that allow the fit to be more customized to your body shape and size (Figure 49, left).

A silicone prosthesis can be heavy, especially for larger-breasted women, and you may find it tiring. But the balanced weight it provides helps to keep your shoulders even and your posture straight. This makes it easier on your neck and shoulder.

Prices for silicone prostheses range from under $100 to about $500 for high-quality products. For public (uninsured) patients in Australia and the UK, prostheses are free, at least for the first one. In the US, some states govern that insurance companies need to provide at least some reimbursement. Check with your insurer or government program to learn what help is available to you. Many private insurance companies pay for a breast prosthesis and a bra. In the US, Medicare will not pay for any bra

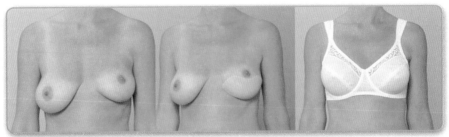

Figure 50: A smaller partial prosthesis, sometimes useful after breast conservation.

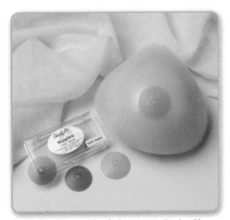

Figure 51: An example of a breast prosthesis with optional stick-on nipple.

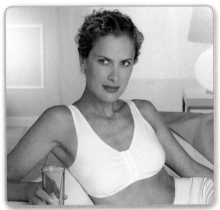

Figure 52: Front-closing cotton bras with pockets are best just after your surgery and during radiotherapy.

unless it has a built in pocket produced at the manufacturer. Medicare allows one silicone breast prosthesis form every two years based on medical necessity. Six mastectomy bras every year are also usually allowed. Medicare usually pays for a camisole immediately following surgery, and one lightweight form every six months is normally covered.

In Australia, from 1 July 2008, an external prosthesis is reimbursable up to $A800 every two years for two sides or $400 for one side. For more information see:

www.medicareaustralia.gov.au/public/files/2231-fact-sheet.pdf

There are also special smaller prostheses for women who have had breast conservation surgery. These may be worn inside the bra and are shaped to fill out a small part of the breast (Figure 50). They are made of the same silicone material as most full-breast prostheses. Some have a stick-on backing.

Nipples can be added to prostheses if required (Figure 51). Swimsuits and lingerie designed for women who have had mastectomies are available by catalog from Lands' End, Sears, Nordstrom, and JC Penney in the USA; and Myer and David Jones in Australia; as well as in small shops and department stores in several countries.

The clothing comes with a pocket to hold the prosthesis. You can also have pockets sewn into the bras or swimsuits you already own.

You should be able to wear a normal bra with a prosthesis. The bra should fit well and offer medium to firm control. You could get a pocket sewn into your bra or sew two ribbons across the inside to hold the prosthesis. Wearing a soft cotton bra that opens at the front with a soft-form prosthesis is a good way to start, particularly if your arm is restricted after surgery to the armpit (Figure 52).

These bras, available from most major manufacturers who specialize in post-breast surgery products, have pockets in both cups to fit a soft-form prosthesis. The soft cotton helps with any discomfort associated with your scar. They are also very good during radiotherapy not only because you can get them off quickly for your daily treatment but also because these bras are relatively inexpensive so it's no problem if you get any of the skin marks from your radiotherapy on the bra.

There are also some very practical and attractive bras and swimwear that are designed to hold a prosthesis (Figures 53 and 54). Make sure you get an appointment for a fitting for your prosthesis. Don't be rushed into making your choice.

Look at and try on as many as possible and be sure that the one you buy comes with a 12-month warranty. When you go for a fitting, take a shirt, blouse, and/or t-shirt so that you can see the final result.

Check that the prosthesis fills your bra cup at both the top and the bottom. A softer silicone prosthesis will give a more natural shape. Stand upright and check in the mirror for shape and a good match to your natural breast. Swing your arms back and forth to check that the form is not too full under your arm.

Care of your prosthesis

Most prostheses, properly cared for, last two to three years. Ensure that you:

- hand wash your prosthesis regularly, preferably daily
- store the prosthesis in the box it came in to help it keep its shape
- avoid wearing a silicone-filled prosthesis in a saltwater or chlorinated pool or in a heated sauna or spa, as it may heat up against your skin

The ideal bra after a mastectomy

The Breast Cancer Care Organization in the UK has published some excellent guidelines called "A Confident Choice, Breast Prostheses, Bras And Clothes—Tips And Advice After Surgery." Their advice states that a proper bra should have:

- Good separation between the cups, which should not be too low

- Good depth under the arm with a lower cut to avoid rubbing and an under-band (below cups) at least 10 mm deep

- A firm or elasticized upper edge to the cups and good straps

- Full cups to cover the prosthesis

- At least two hooks to fasten at the back (more in larger sizes)

Also look for a bra that is wider under the arm so there is greater support around the back and to cover any scars or areas of puckering around your scar. Most of these features can be seen below and can be found at:

www.breastcancercare.org.uk/content.php?page_id=3487

At first, it's a good idea to buy just one bra (or at most two bras), in case it turns out to be unsuitable—for example, if it's not comfortable or the cup doesn't cover the prosthesis well enough, or in case your bra size changes with changes in your

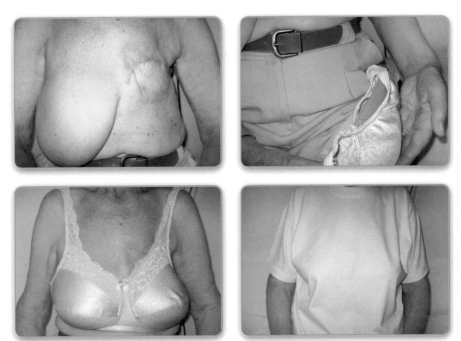

Figure 53: Use of an external breast prosthesis inserted into a custom bra slip.

weight as a result of your treatment. You could keep the bra in its packaging until you have your prosthesis fitting so that you can change it if you need to. Judi Simon, President and CEO of Nearly Me Technologies, Inc., said "that the longevity of any bra, fashion or mastectomy, is only 16 washings. Because of the use of synthetic fibers, all bras lose their elasticity and support after that amount of wear. This seems to be standard across the lingerie industry. Also, hand washing versus machine washing and drying prolongs the life of the garment. We always recommend to our patients that they purchase at least three bras at a time (one in the wash, one to wear, and one as a spare).

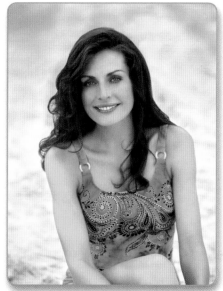

Figure 54: Specialized swimwear with adjustable shoulder straps and a special bust with pockets on both sides to allow a breast prosthesis.

Also, it is highly recommended that they go back to their fitter every six months, since if they gain or lose even ten pounds, it will change the look and weight of the remaining natural breast and therefore how the prosthesis fits and mimics their body."

CONTROL POINT #5 – IF I HAVE A MASTECTOMY, CAN I WEAR AN EXTERNAL PROSTHESIS?

WARNING After breast surgery, and also after radiation therapy, your chest area can be extra sensitive, so it's best to delay getting an external silicone prosthesis until about eight weeks after treatment is completed.

TIP Wearing a soft cotton bra that opens at the front with a soft-form prosthesis is a good way to start after your surgery, particularly if your arm is restricted or you are having radiation therapy.

REMEMBER Talk to your bra and prosthesis fitter or breast care nurse about your options for a bra or prosthesis sooner rather than later after your surgery.

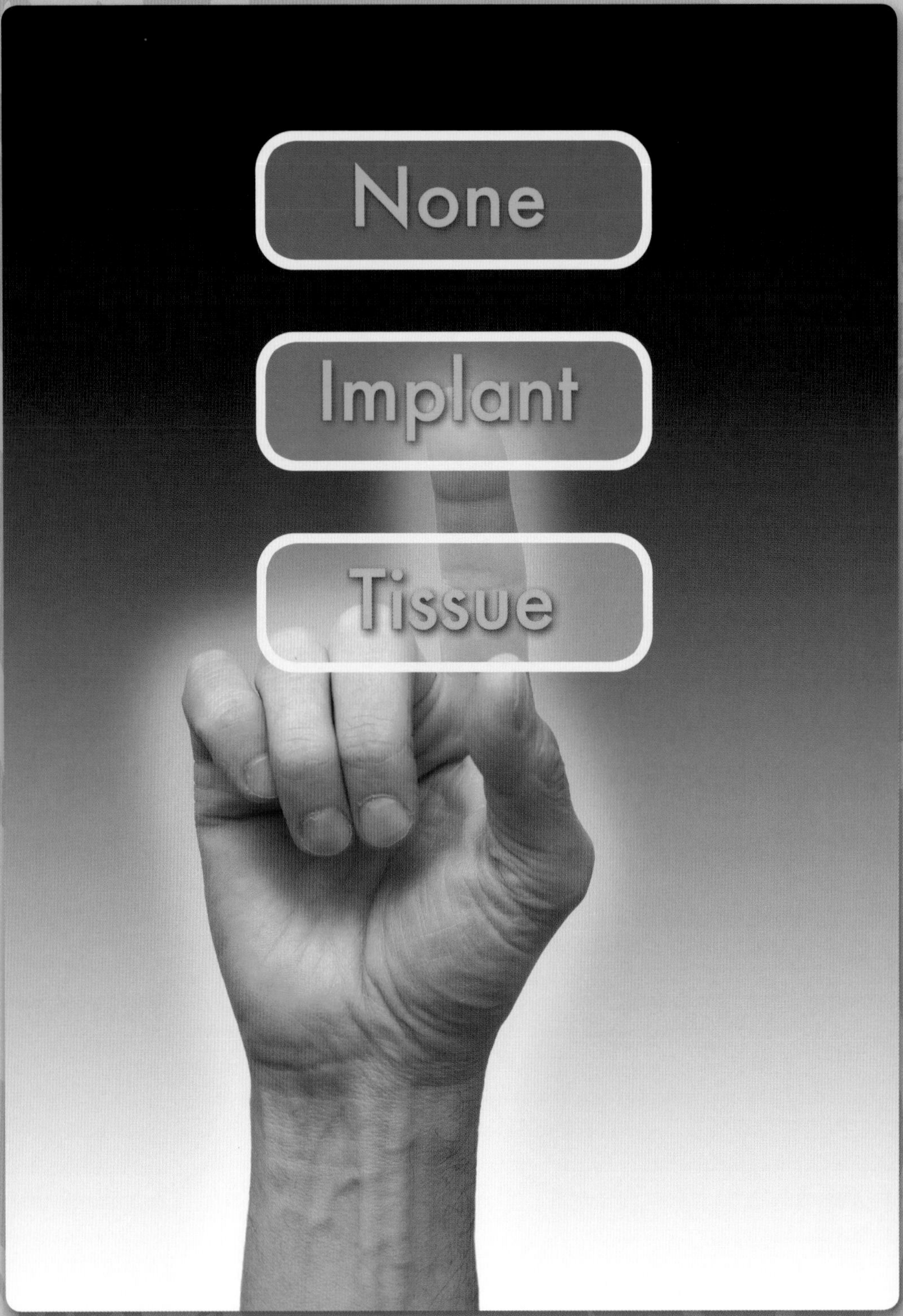
None
Implant
Tissue

Control Point 6

What Are My Options for Breast Reconstruction?

Control Point #6

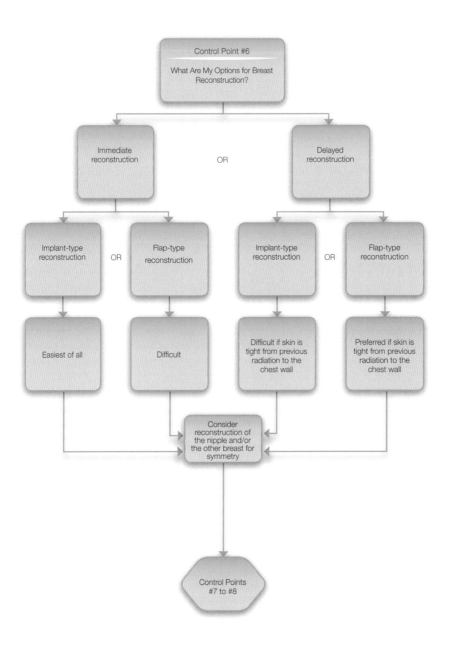

Control Point #6

What Are My Options for Breast Reconstruction?

Immediate reconstruction **OR** Delayed reconstruction

Implant-type reconstruction **OR** Flap-type reconstruction

Implant-type reconstruction **OR** Flap-type reconstruction

Easiest of all

Difficult

Difficult if skin is tight from previous radiation to the chest wall

Preferred if skin is tight from previous radiation to the chest wall

Consider reconstruction of the nipple and/or the other breast for symmetry

Control Points #7 to #8

6

What Are My Options for Breast Reconstruction?

Having a breast reconstruction is a very personal decision and you should not be pressured one way or another by your partner, friends, or doctors. Take control of this decision by getting as much information as you can from your treating doctors; support groups; organizations, and if possible, other women who have gone through the same procedure.

Don't feel rushed by your surgeon's operating schedule; take the time to work out the best option for you right now. This could include never having a reconstruction, having it done in a few years (**delayed reconstruction**), or having it at the same time as your mastectomy (**immediate reconstruction**). If you're having an immediate reconstruction, the plastic surgeon will usually take over directly after the mastectomy, while you're still under anesthetic. Some surgeons are trained to do both the mastectomy and a more limited type of reconstruction which is often referred to as oncoplastic surgery.

There are many myths about having a breast reconstruction after a mastectomy, but one thing that's certain is that it's a complex decision. Factors that influence this decision include not only your thoughts and feelings, but also the availability of expertise and resources, such as your specialist team and the availability of operating theater time.

What is breast reconstruction?

Breast reconstruction is a complex procedure, and often, you may need two or more operations to achieve a correctly positioned new breast. However, your breasts probably won't be completely symmetrical afterward and will never be like your own natural breast. Still, many women choose to have reconstructions. Different approaches to breast reconstruction include:

• Using tissue expanders and breast implants

• Using your body's own tissue ("tissue" or "flap" reconstruction)

• Using a combination of tissue reconstruction and implants.

Understand what breast reconstruction surgery can do for you, but also be aware of what it won't do for you. It will involve more surgery that takes longer under the anesthetic than surgery without a reconstruction, and that is associated with more side effects, but it will give you a "mound," either constructed from your own tissue or using a silicone implant.

The breast reconstruction process can also include reconstruction of your nipple, but some women omit this step because the reconstructed nipple is only cosmetic and will not function like your natural nipple.

Finally, you may choose to have surgery on your other breast, even if it's healthy, so that it more closely matches the shape and size of your reconstructed breast. This can, for example, involve an enhancement, or more usually a "lift" (mastopexy) or a reduction, particularly if you had large breasts to start with.

When can I have breast reconstruction?

If you think you may want a breast reconstruction, it's very important to discuss this with your breast surgeon before your breast cancer operation. Ask your breast surgeon to arrange an appointment with a plastic surgeon before your mastectomy to discuss whether or not you are more suited to an immediate reconstruction, a delayed reconstruction, or no reconstruction.

You may want to see one or two reconstructive surgeons who work with your breast surgeon. It may be best to see one who has experience in all types of reconstructions, including implants and non-implant procedures using your own tissue. Ask to see some photographs of their work, or better still, see if you can talk to one or two of their previous patients.

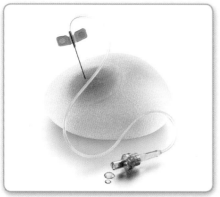 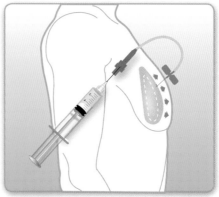

Figure 55: Pictured above is an expander, to be inserted behind the pectoralis major muscle. Saltwater is injected into its magnetic port (at tip of green butterfly needle) once a week for roughly four to six weeks.

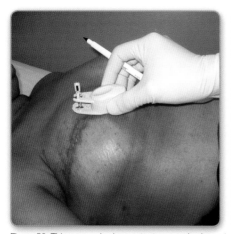 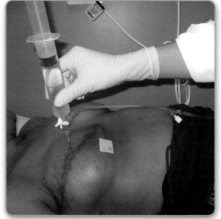

Figure 56: This woman had a mastectomy and sub-pectoral implant. A magnet (left) is used to find the exact location of the port under the skin. A needle and syringe full of saline (right) is then used to inflate the implant at regular intervals.

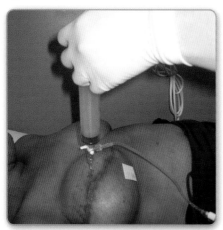 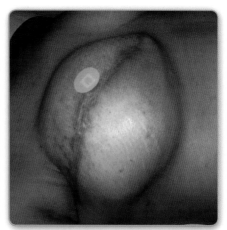

Figure 57: A further 50 mL of saline was inserted into the implant before the patient's radiation treatment started.

What Are My Options for Breast Reconstruction?   121

Most oncologists can normally work out the timing of treatments such as chemotherapy and hormonal treatment with a reconstruction. Common approaches to timing are shown in Figure 86.

Ultimately, your own feelings, thoughts, and instincts are critical. Take control here and don't be rushed. It may take a few extra days to get all the information you need.

Different types of breast reconstruction

Tissue expansion and breast implants

A breast implant is a round or teardrop-shaped silicone shell that's filled with saline or silicone gel. A plastic surgeon places the implant behind the muscle in your chest (pectoral muscle) in a manner similar to that which occurs during breast augmentation (enlargement) surgery (Figure 55). Sometimes, a mastectomy is done on both sides and bilateral implants are inserted, particularly if there is a strong family history of breast cancer.

Few women are able to go through a one-stage implantation process—receiving the final, permanent implant at the time of the mastectomy. Rather, most women require a two-stage process, using a temporary **tissue expander** before the permanent implant is placed. Tissue expansion involves stretching your remaining chest skin and soft tissues to make room for the breast implant. After the tissue expander is implanted, you'll need to visit your doctor's office every week or two, for a total of five or six visits, to have small amounts of saltwater (saline) inserted into the expander through a magnetic port. The port is magnetic so that the nurse or doctor can use a magnet to quickly find the access port and inject the saline. It's a bit like a beach balloon that slowly gets inflated with saline rather than air (Figure 56).

The skin is stretched slowly to avoid too much discomfort or pressure as the implant expands, but some minor discomfort is often associated with the procedure (Figure 57). The first day or so after your surgery is usually when you'll be the most uncomfortable.

After the tissue expansion process is complete, your surgeon will perform further surgery to remove the tissue expander and replace it with a permanent implant, which has a more natural look and feel. This normally takes place six to nine months after the implant is first inserted. Once complete, the final result can look very good in a bra (Figure 58). Over time, implants may rupture or need replacement. However, implants involve less surgery, less pain, shorter recovery, no additional scar, and less expense than **flap reconstruction**.

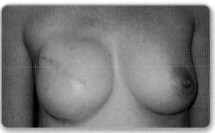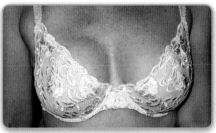

Figure 58: A mound has been produced that looks good in a bra.

Although an implant reconstruction may be performed at the same time as your mastectomy, or at a later time, it cannot usually be performed after radiation therapy is given to the chest area after a mastectomy (**post-mastectomy radiation therapy**). This is because radiation treatment can cause tightening and reduced flexibility or stretch of the skin, making the implant impossible to insert (Figure 59). Sometimes, though, it can be done if there is some stretch left in the skin. If radiation therapy is necessary, a flap reconstruction is preferable if a delayed reconstruction is done because the irradiated skin can be removed and replaced with healthy skin from another part of the body (a **"donor site"**).

Radiation after a mastectomy will be covered later, but the main reasons it's usually given are because your cancer has spread to four or more lymph glands under your armpit, or the cancer is larger than 50 mm (about 2 inches) or larger.

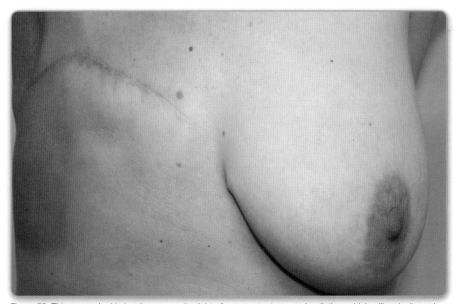

Figure 59: This woman's skin has become quite tight after a mastectomy and radiation, which will make it nearly impossible to have a sub-pectoral implant reconstruction. A "flap" reconstruction will be required instead.

Tissue or flap reconstruction

This is the most complex reconstructive option, but it has the advantage of a more natural look and feel. With tissue or flap reconstruction, your surgeon moves a section of skin, muscle, fat, and blood vessels from one part of your body to your chest to create a new breast mound. The nipple can be recreated later. Flap reconstructions require three to eight hours of surgery, and sometimes longer.

Because muscle flap reconstruction requires healthy blood vessels, women with diabetes, connective tissue disease, vascular disease, previous major abdominal surgery, or a history of smoking may need to consider other options.

During a flap reconstruction, flaps of muscle and skin are taken from the back, abdomen, or buttocks. In some cases, the skin and tissue need to be expanded further with a breast implant to achieve the desired breast size.

Flaps can be "free" or "attached" from the donor source and original blood supply. A **free flap** means that the "flap" of skin, fat, and muscle tissue is completely detached and then connected to a new supply of blood vessels in the original breast area without tunneling under the skin. The surgeon detaches the tissue completely from its blood supply and uses microsurgery to reattach the tissue flap to new blood vessels near your chest. Because of the intricate nature of reattaching blood vessels using microsurgery, free flap surgery typically takes longer to complete than pedicle flap surgery does.

Not all plastic surgeons can do microsurgery. The free flap procedure can have a higher complication rate, so make sure that you see a highly skilled specialist. However, many surgeons believe that the free flap allows them to create a more natural shape than the attached or pedicle flap.

An attached or "pedicle" flap is tunneled under the skin whilst the flap is connected to the original donor source and blood supply. There are four common types of flap reconstructions: latissimus dorsi, TRAM, DIEP, and gluteal.

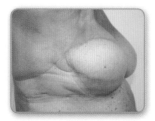 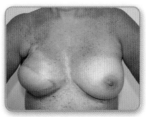 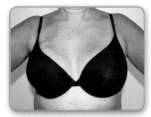

Figure 60: Different views of a latissimus dorsi muscle flap. A sub-pectoral implant was also inserted on the left side to match the size of the new breast on the right side.

The **latissimus dorsi muscle flap** is taken from the back, with its own blood supply, and is tunneled under the skin to the front of the chest (Figure 60). The flap is not large, and it may therefore be necessary to use a small implant as well as the flap. This is a useful technique if you do not have large breasts or if previous abdominal surgery prevents using abdominal tissue.

The **transverse rectus abdominus muscle (TRAM) flap** procedure uses tissue tunneled from your lower abdomen—including a full thickness of skin, fat, and muscle—that is either attached to its own blood supply (or "pedicle") or detached ("free") from its own blood supply. This muscle flap will create a reconstructed breast at the mastectomy site with no areola or nipple (Figure 61). It also means that some of the fat and muscle in your abdomen is used, so a "tummy tuck" is an added bonus. The downside is that there can be more weakness in the abdomen, and a hernia is a possible complication. There is no doubt that this is a major procedure, and it can take many weeks to fully recover, but most women are happy with the very natural feel of their new breast. Although the scars in Figure 61 look prominent, they will fade and be less visible within four to six months of surgery.

The **deep inferior epigastric perforator (DIEP) flap** abdominal procedure uses blood vessels in the abdomen that travel through (perforate) the rectus abdominus muscle to supply the overlying abdominal skin. This newer procedure is almost the same as a TRAM flap, but skin and fat are the only tissues removed, so no muscle is taken. The flap uses a free (detached) flap approach, which allows you to retain more strength in your abdomen. If your surgeon can't perform a DIEP flap procedure

for anatomical reasons, he or she might opt instead for the muscle-sparing free TRAM flap. Studies have shown that there are fewer abdominal complications from the DIEP flap because muscle is not taken. The **superficial inferior epigastric artery (SIEA) flap** is very similar but uses different blood vessels.

A good website for more information is www.microsurgeon.org

The British Association of Plastic Reconstructive and Aesthetic Surgeons is also useful: www.bapras.org.uk/

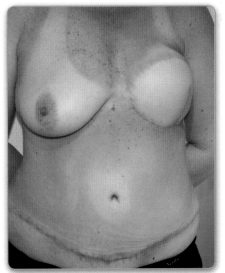

Figure 61: About three months after a TRAM flap with no nipple reconstruction, showing the new breast and the scar in the lower abdomen (the donor site).

The **gluteal (or buttock) flap** is a free flap procedure that takes tissue—possibly including muscle—from your buttocks and transplants it to your chest area after the mastectomy is finished. There are two forms of gluteal flaps: the S-GAP, or "superior gluteal artery perforator," reconstruction uses tissue from the top of the buttock, which contains the upper gluteal artery. I-GAP, or "inferior gluteal artery perforator," uses tissue taken from the crease of the buttock (where the buttocks meet the thigh) that contains the lower gluteal artery. A rounded section of skin and fat (and occasionally muscle) is removed either from the top of the buttock or the crease along the underside of the buttock. After being transferred to the breast, the tissue is shaped to create the breast mound and is attached to the remaining breast tissue using microsurgery. It can take several weeks to recover from such a procedure and there will be scars in the buttocks area and the breast that will need to heal. There may be noticeable asymmetry between the buttocks after the flap is taken. Antibiotics are often given before and after surgery to reduce the risk of infection. Table 2 below summarizes the different types of flap reconstructions.

Nipple reconstruction

Not all women choose to have nipple reconstruction. It's entirely up to you. Some women can't really be bothered going back for surgery and it's perfectly okay if you feel that way. The nipple can also be reconstructed and tattooed to reproduce an appropriate color match with your other breast. The reconstructed nipple will not have sensation. Silicone "stick-on" nipples are also available.

Nipple reconstruction is usually done in one of two ways: your surgeon can use the skin of your reconstruction, raising it and bringing it together to look like a nipple; or "nipple sharing" by transferring part of your nipple from the other side (Figure 62). The areola is reconstructed by using a skin graft, usually from the crease of your groin, or is simply tattooed. Neither method will give you a functioning, sensitive nipple; reconstruction is strictly cosmetic.

Flap	Latissimus Dorsi	TRAM (pedicle)	TRAM (free)	DIEP	Gluteal
Type of Flap	Pedicle	Pedicle	Free	Free	Free
Donor Site	Upper back	Abdomen	Abdomen	Abdomen	Buttock
Muscle Removed	Yes	Yes	Yes	No	Yes
Suitable with Previous Abdominal Surgery	Definite	Possible	Possible	Possible	Definite
Microsurgery Needed	No	No	Yes	Yes	Yes
Procedure Time (hrs)	2–4	6–8	6–8	6–8	8–12
Days in Hospital	4	7	7	7	7
Smaller Breasted	Yes	Yes	Yes	Yes	Yes
Larger Breasted	Yes, with implant	Yes	Yes	Yes	Yes
Chance of Flap Breakdown or "Necrosis"	Not common	Often minor wound healing problems and partial flap loss	< 5% total flap loss	< 5% total flap loss	< 8% total flap loss
Chance of Abdominal Hernia	No	Yes (<5%)	Yes (<2%)	Yes (<1%)	No
Sensation	No nipple	No nipple	No nipple	No nipple	No nipple

Table 2: Comparison between different types of flap reconstructions

Reconstruction of your other breast

Sometimes your plastic surgeon will talk to you about the other breast. Inevitably, your other breast will not be the same as your reconstructed breast in terms of size and position. Surgery to the other breast can improve symmetry.

This may be a "lift," or mastopexy or a reduction known as a **reduction mammoplasty** (Figure 62), or even an implant to enlarge the other side (Figure 60). Removal of the other breast (prophylactic mastectomy) is very rarely considered, though we may discuss it if you have an exceptionally strong family history of breast cancer and you feel it's easier to have just one anesthetic, remove the burden of constant mammography on that side, and ensure a symmetrical reconstruction. However, don't rush this decision—it takes a lot of thought and discussion. Always make sure that your plastic surgeon sends any normal tissue from the reduced side for examination by the pathologist.

Recovery after a reconstruction

You are likely to feel quite tired and sore for a week or two after implant reconstruction, and for up to three to six weeks after flap procedures. Most of your discomfort can be controlled by painkillers prescribed by your doctor. You'll also have stitches (sutures) in place after your surgery. They'll probably be the kind that dissolve on their own, so you won't need to have them removed.

Depending on the type of surgery, you should be able to leave hospital in one to ten days. Surgical drains are used to remove fluid from the site of your operation. Usually, these drains are removed while you're in the hospital, but sometimes you can be discharged with a drain still in place.

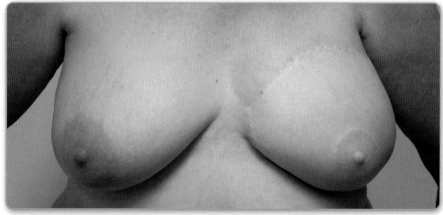

Figure 62: A left TRAM flap reconstruction with a nipple reconstruction and a reduction of the right side for balance.

Follow your surgeon's advice on stretching exercises and returning to your normal activities. Getting back to normal activities may take up to six weeks or more, depending on the type of procedure performed. Take it easy during this period. Your doctor will let you know of any restrictions to your activities, such as avoiding overhead lifting or strenuous physical activities. Don't be surprised if it seems to take a long time to bounce back from surgery.

If you've had one breast reconstructed, you'll need to have a screening mammogram done regularly for your other breast. Mammography isn't done on your reconstructed breast, but a CT, MRI, or ultrasound may be done if we ever need to look behind your reconstruction. You may opt to perform breast self-exams on your natural breast and on the skin and surrounding area of your reconstructed breast. If cancer comes back on the reconstructed side, it usually appears as small "pimples" or nodules, often around your scar.

Complications and risks of a reconstruction

Breast reconstruction carries the possibility of complications. Most commonly, expanders will feel tight until the surrounding tissue stretches. Further, breast implants aren't lifelong devices, and you may eventually need surgery to replace or remove the implant. Also, with breast implants, you could experience complications such as infection or rotation (where the implant moves into the wrong position).

There is a slightly higher risk of infection around the implant with chemotherapy, and an increased risk of **capsulitis**, or capsular contracture. Capsulitis is when scar tissue forms and compresses the implant into a hard and unnatural shape. The odds of this occurring increase in the 12 to 24 months after you have had radiation therapy to the chest wall and implant. These complications may require additional surgery.

Tissue reconstruction is a major procedure. It prolongs your time in surgery and can extend your recovery time by several weeks. Flaps cause pain both at the "donor" site and in the chest area. Removal of muscles from the donor site will cause pain and weakness, or rarely, a hernia.

In addition, poor wound healing, a hernia in your abdominal scar, a collection of fluid (seroma), and/or infection can occur. The worst complication, which is rare, is when the flap doesn't take due to tissue death (a bit like gangrene) from insufficient blood supply. Complications are more common if you are overweight, have diabetes, or are a smoker.

Should I have breast reconstruction?

Some women find a mastectomy without reconstruction a constant reminder of their cancer. There is some evidence from the UK and the US that you may feel more positive about yourself if you have a reconstruction after a mastectomy.

Nevertheless, many women are quite comfortable not having a reconstruction and feel relieved that their cancer has been removed and the breast is gone. I sometimes hear surgeons saying, "Forget the reconstruction for now because we don't want to delay your cancer treatment," but this is a misinformed statement. Your cancer has probably been there for many months, and perhaps even a year or so in some circumstances. A few days' or even a few weeks' delay in getting treatments that generally take place after surgery will not change your prognosis at all.

Your general health, previous abdominal treatments (which can affect the donor area for a flap reconstruction), and your proposed cancer treatment are taken into account to work out which type of reconstruction will give you the best result. The plastic surgeon will give you information on the anesthesia, the location of the operation, and what kind of follow-up procedures may be necessary.

In Australia, for example, less than five percent of women have access to an immediate reconstruction, usually because of a lack of expertise and the logistical difficulties of having a breast surgeon operate at the same time as the plastic surgeon. At our group of hospitals, all women are offered a reconstruction, but only about 40 percent take up the offer after a full and frank discussion.

Some women prefer to think about an immediate reconstruction whereas others really just want to have a mastectomy and think about a reconstruction a year or two later. There is no correct answer. Go with not only what is available to you but also with what you feel comfortable doing at this stage. You can always reconsider a reconstruction at a later time.

It's important to understand what you can expect from a breast reconstruction before you make your decision. A reconstruction will not give you a new, normally functioning breast. The difference between your reconstructed and your natural breast will be minimal when you're dressed but usually obvious when you're undressed. Having a reconstruction will provide a contour or shape so that you'll be able to wear most of your usual clothes and swimwear.

In summary, don't be rushed by your surgeon about this very important decision. It's far better to delay your surgery a week or two and get the right advice than it is to try to conform with your surgeon's operating schedule. Let him or her panic, rather than you, while you get some sound advice.

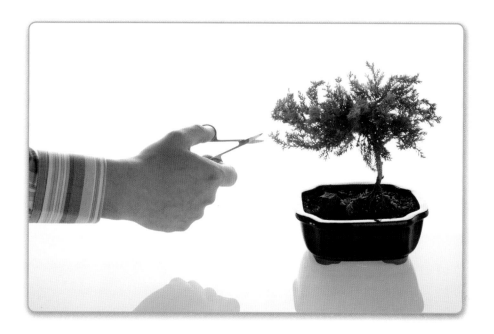

CONTROL POINT #6 – WHAT ARE MY OPTIONS FOR BREAST RECONSTRUCTION?

WARNING
An implant reconstruction cannot usually be performed after radiation therapy is given to the chest area. If your doctor feels that there is a chance you will need radiation to the chest wall after a mastectomy, ask to see a plastic surgeon before your surgery.

TIP
Don't feel rushed by your surgeon's operating schedule; take the time to work out the best option for you right now. This could include never having a reconstruction, having it done in a few years (delayed reconstruction), or having it done at the same time as your mastectomy (immediate reconstruction).

REMEMBER
Having a breast reconstruction is a very personal decision and you should not be pressured one way or another by your partner, friends, or doctors.

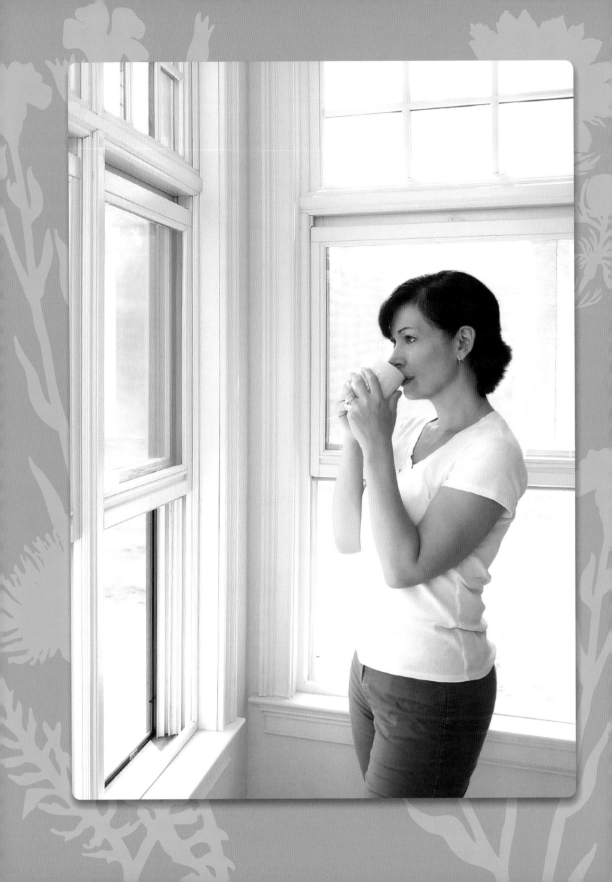

Control Point 7

What Should I Do before I Go into the Hospital?

Control Point #7

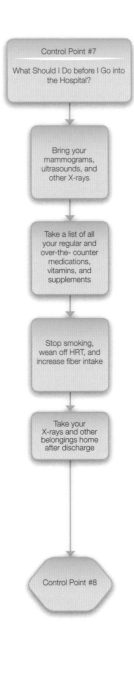

Control Point #7

What Should I Do before I Go into the Hospital?

Bring your mammograms, ultrasounds, and other X-rays

Take a list of all your regular and over-the- counter medications, vitamins, and supplements

Stop smoking, wean off HRT, and increase fiber intake

Take your X-rays and other belongings home after discharge

Control Point #8

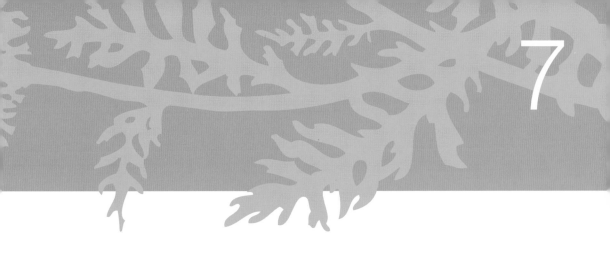

7

What Should I Do before I Go into the Hospital?

Tips before you go into the hospital

Going into the hospital, particularly for the first time, can be frightening and overwhelming. This control point will give you some ideas to make your hospital stay a little easier. Your doctor or nurse will also give you specific information about the hospital you'll be going to.

- Stop smoking as soon as possible. Speak to your doctor about nicotine gum or patches to combat cravings and urges to smoke.

- Eat well before you go into the hospital; take fiber, because you can get constipated lying around in a hospital bed

- Take a list of all your regular medications and over-the-counter preparations

- Pack toiletries, including toothbrush, soap, shampoo, aluminum-free deodorant, and face wipes. Aluminum is thought to make skin reaction from radiation therapy worse.

- Bring details of past illnesses (dates and diagnoses) and a list of allergies

- Pack makeup and a hair dryer if desired

- Take glasses or contact lenses and eye drops if needed

- Pack slippers, a comfy robe, and pajamas if staying for more than one day. Button-up pajamas are slightly more practical than night gowns.

- Take photos of family or loved ones

- Take your pillow, quilt cover, or perhaps a familiar cushion or a throw rug for the visitor's chair

- Bring cash for phone calls, the coffee shop, etc. but leave jewelry at home

- Take your health cards (e.g. Medicare or insurance card) and the name, address, and contact numbers of your family doctor and specialist

- Leave jewelry at home

- Bring your mammograms, ultrasounds, and other X-rays (but don't forget to take them home with you!)

- Bring any hospital identification cards or record numbers

- Pack reading material, such as books and magazines

- Bring your mobile phone and portable computer (and DVDs if you'll have a long stay), and don't forget your power cords and chargers

- Take a couple of bottles of your favorite water because the hospital air conditioning can dry out your throat

- Pack your portable music player if you have one

- Don't forget your telephone and address book or PDA

- Take a power strip if you have lots of electronic equipment

- Stop taking aspirin, the pill, hormone (replacement) therapy, and green tea, as these can influence clotting (talk to your team to see what they advise)

- If you are a diabetic, be diligent about monitoring your sugar levels before going into the hospital

- Find out what time to arrive, where to go, and how long you need to fast beforehand

- Get details on the costs of treatment, including the specialist, anesthetist, pathologist, and hospital fees.

Tips when you arrive into the hospital

When you arrive in the hospital for the first time you will to check in at the admissions office which is usually near the main entrance.

Work out how to use the:

- call system between you and the nurse

- telephones and the bed controls

Find out about:

- access you might have to television, radio, newspapers, or the Internet
- access you might have to storage of any valuables
- the hospital's visitor policy and visiting times, and where your visitors can park
- when you can expect to be discharged and at what time.

It's not unusual to feel weak or tired while in the hospital, so use the call button when you need help. Be careful not to trip over wires or tubes when you get in or out of bed. It's best to keep your things within easy reach. Make sure you hold onto support bars when getting in or out of the bath or shower, and use the handrails on stairways and in hallways. Most doctors and hospitals now encourage early mobilization to get your feet and legs moving to prevent blood clots.

Tips for the elderly

Hospital stays can be quite disorienting, particularly for the elderly. when removed from their usual environment. If you are a family member reading this, please be aware that older people (particularly over 75–80) can drift from being relatively independent to dependent in a surprisingly short period of time. You can help by bringing familiar things to the hospital such as family photos or a favorite pillow or gown. A strange hospital ward can be a very frightening place for the elderly, and you may need to stay overnight with them. Find out how this can be done if required.

CONTROL POINT #7 – WHAT SHOULD I DO BEFORE I GO INTO THE HOSPITAL

 WARNING Stop smoking as soon as possible. Eat well before you go into the hospital; take fiber, because you can get constipated lying around in a hospital bed.

 TIP Take a list of all your regular medications and over-the-counter preparations.

 REMEMBER Bring your mammograms, ultrasounds, and other X-rays, and don't forget to take them home with you.

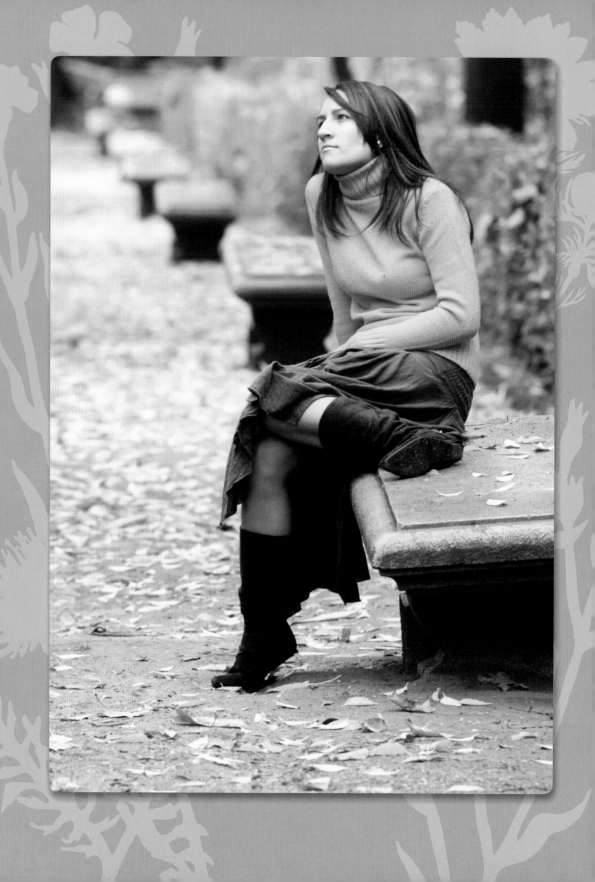

Control Point 8

How Do I Cope with Waiting for My Results?

Control Point #8

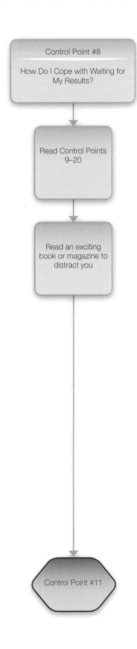

Control Point #8

How Do I Cope with Waiting for My Results?

Read Control Points 9–20

Read an exciting book or magazine to distract you

Control Point #11

8

How Do I Cope with Waiting for My Results?

Tips while waiting for your results

The week after your surgery will be one of those really bad weeks. I mentioned above that waiting to see the doctor for the first time is a horrible week. Well, this week, waiting around for the results, is even worse. You may be in a state of shock. You may have been rushed into surgery without enough time to get your thoughts and your information together.

Your results will take a while to come through. If you're up to it, start getting your thoughts together before you leave the hospital, and start reading Part 3 of this book if you have not already done so. Take some control at this point by getting ready for your next doctor's appointment.

A good doctor will talk to you like a real human being and try to give you as much time as possible. That's the good news. The flip side is that they're doing that with all their other patients too, so they'll battle to run their appointments on time. This can be frustrating. Doctors who treat breast cancer usually do not run on time, as it's often unpredictable and difficult to know if a patient will take 30 to 60 minutes or five minutes. In addition, they may have one or two "urgent" cases squeezed onto their list, which makes the waiting times worse.

Like you, other patients will be getting their results on the same day that you are, and most people will have lots of questions. Just as with the doctor, the receptionist often can't predict how long things will take.

Waiting to get your results after your surgery is not only scary, but also very frustrating, and you may feel you are waiting to receive your "sentence." You may experience periods of depression, anger, and hurt as you worry over questions like: Will it be good news or not so good? Will I need chemotherapy? Do I have any hope?

Here are some hints to help you cope:

- Talk to your family, friends, and children about your surgery and your feelings

- Do not be afraid to show your husband or partner your scar, even if you've had a mastectomy. This is a really important but often difficult step for emotional healing.

- Get ready for your post-operative doctor's visit. Have your questions ready and, importantly, written down. I have some key questions you can ask at the back of this book. Make sure you take that checklist when you see your doctor.

- You may find that you receive conflicting advice from different nurses or junior doctors on the ward about how to manage your scar, so do not be afraid to ask your surgeon directly about his or her preferred method

- Keep reading your favorite novel or book or get back on your computer and keep in touch with the outside world. When you go to your doctor's office, take a book or magazine to read, or some craftwork if you are that way inclined or your iPod, to keep you occupied while you wait.

- If you're a person who likes researching your own condition, exercise caution regarding how much information you seek out online. There's a wealth of information out there, but not all of it is good or even right. Some of it will have the potential to scare you or lead you down the wrong path.

- Start walking and try to build up to half an hour a day, three or four times a week

- Start on a healthy diet, but don't be afraid to have the odd bit of chocolate or treat as a reward, maybe at the end of the week

- When you have reasonable shoulder movement (and if you have power steering), take yourself for a short drive

- If you're not taking pain medication, small amounts (one or at most two glasses a day) of alcohol are okay.

Being prepared when you see your surgeon

Here is a checklist you can take with you to your appointment to help remind you of everything you should ask your doctor:

- Is there any sign of redness or pain around the scar to suggest infection? If there is, consider taking an antibiotic for a week.

- How much fluid has been draining daily out of the drain in your armpit? Keep an accurate record of the daily amount. This will help your surgeon determine whether to take out the drain at your next visit or whether you may need to come back a second time.

- Be sure you ask the surgeon for a copy of the pathology report

- Ask your surgeon to highlight these important findings:

  - The size of the tumor in millimeters or inches

  - The type of cancer (e.g. invasive ductal, lobular, tubular, etc.)

  - The margin of normal tissue around the tumor

  - The **histologic grade** of the tumor

  - The number of lymph glands removed by your surgeon

  - The number of lymph glands found with cancer

There are a number of test results that are not available straight away and may take an extra few days or a week to come back. These tests are fairly critical for making decisions about **adjuvant**, or additional, therapy over and above the surgery.

These tests are:

- The **estrogen receptor** test (and to a lesser extent, the **progesterone receptor** test), which determines if your breast cancer is sensitive to anti-estrogen therapies

- The **HER2 receptor** test, which determines if a drug called **Herceptin** will work against your cancer

- The final immuno-histochemistry test on your sentinel node, particularly if the quick test was clear.

Waiting to see your doctor after your surgery is a very anxious time, as you will naturally be worried about the final pathology results; whether or not you will need more surgery; and what other treatments, specifically radiation therapy, chemotherapy, or hormonal treatment, you will need.

There is a lot to discuss at your first postoperative visit. It's best to bring somebody along with you, and even a person who can take some notes. Control Points #9 to #19 are the key decisions and steps that you and your doctor will need to think about after your surgery to work out the best treatment—not for some theoretical person in a textbook, but for you and your own individual circumstances.

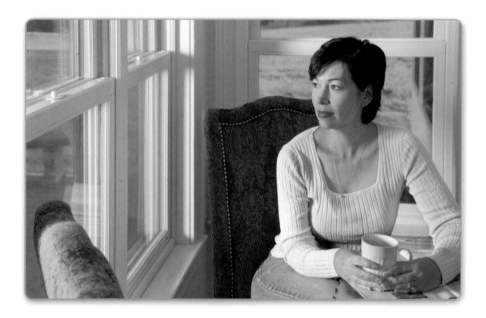

CONTROL POINT #8 – HOW DO I COPE WITH WAITING FOR MY RESULTS?

WARNING If you're a person who likes researching your own condition, exercise caution regarding how much information you seek out online. There's a wealth of information out there, but not all of it is good or even right.

TIP Keep reading your favorite novel or book or get back on your computer and keep in touch with the outside world. When you go to your doctor's office, take a book or magazine to read, or some craftwork if you are that way inclined, to keep you occupied while you wait.

REMEMBER Talk to your family, friends, and children about your surgery and your feelings.

Kimberley's Story

This was a really difficult time. Waiting for the results was excruciating because there was nothing that I could do but sit and think about the possibility that the news might be the worst.

It seemed to me that I dripped fear from every pore in my body, and I could almost taste it on my breath. Being that afraid worried me too, because I didn't want my body to be enveloped in such negative feelings when I was trying to overcome cancer.

I rang a Cancer Help Line and predictably burst into tears when talking to them. It did help to talk to them, but I was still scared stiff. Then I read some information about dealing with fear. It said that fear was just really strong anxiety and that being afraid didn't actually achieve anything.

That struck a chord with me. I'd learned to listen to fear because it tells us that we are in a dangerous situation and should do something. But here there was no reason to listen to the fear. Everything that could be done was being done and there was nothing I should do.

So I gave myself permission to try my best to ignore my fear. Easier said than done.

I thought about what was the best way to distract myself, and for me that has always been to lose myself in a good book. I hadn't read the Da Vinci Code, and so I immersed myself in that and it worked for me. Occasionally, the fear would flood in, but I would just acknowledge it and say, "Yep, I'm afraid, but it's okay not to think about that," and try to refocus.

Of course I was still afraid, but I felt better that I wasn't afraid all the time.

PART 3

"MAINTAINING CONTROL"

TAKING CONTROL AFTER YOUR SURGERY

Franka's Story

I will always remember seeing a 54-year-old woman with two young children, around October of 2004, who had had a mastectomy for hre left breast 20 years earlier when I was an oncology trainee.

She was told her to put her affairs in order. She'd had 33 lymph glands involved in her armpit. Her prognosis was probably less than 30 percent at ten years.

Twenty years later, she walks in the door with an abnormality in her other breast that turned out to be nothing serious. She was now a grandmother.

This woman clearly showed me that there is always hope, and even if there are a lot of glands involved and the situation appears hopeless at first, it's still important to get the best possible treatment to the breast or chest wall area, the glands, and the rest of the body.

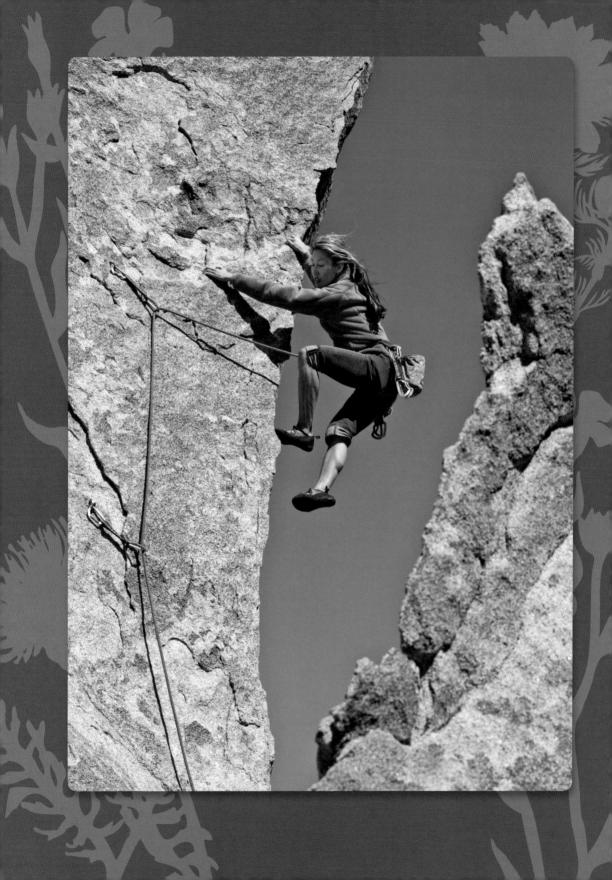

Control Point 9

How Do I Deal With Any Possible Complications?

Control Point #9

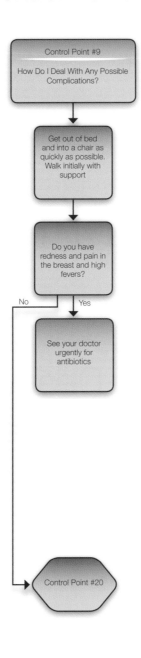

Control Point #9

How Do I Deal With Any Possible Complications?

Get out of bed and into a chair as quickly as possible. Walk initially with support

Do you have redness and pain in the breast and high fevers?

No   Yes

See your doctor urgently for antibiotics

Control Point #20

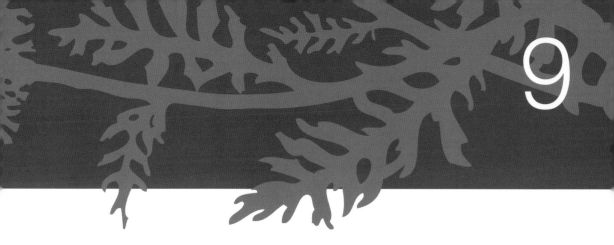

9

How Do I Deal With Any Possible Complications?

Common side effects after surgery

Apart from your emotional wellbeing, coping with your physical side effects and knowing what's normal and what's an unexpected complication of your surgery is really important right now.

The first important step now is to look at the surgical aspects of your breast cancer. The surgeon and oncologist, if you are seeing one, need to check your scars and make sure that there's no infection or bruising. If the lymph glands have been removed, there may be a smaller scar in the armpit, or the same scar from your breast may extend into the armpit (Figure 31). Speak to your surgeon before the surgery to find out exactly how many scars or wounds he or she is planning.

If there's a collection of fluid under the armpit or around the scar in your breast called a seroma, then this will need to be drained. It's a fairly minor procedure that can be done straight away with a needle and syringe by your doctor or nurse. Often the armpit is a little bit numb, and this actually helps lessen the usual stinging you get with an injection.

The wound or wounds will usually be covered by a dressing that can be removed the day after surgery. Underneath the dressing, there may be steri-strips. These are small paper tapes that hold the wound in place and usually come off over the next seven to ten days. If they start to peel, don't get too worried. They can be trimmed using a pair of clean scissors.

I am a big fan of using dissolving stitches under the skin. Some surgeons still use staples or sutures outside the skin, but these are really unnecessary and just cause problems later on with more scarring (Figure 32). The good surgeons know how to place the scars along the natural lines of your skin, which are called **Langer's lines**. Doing so aids healing and yields a better cosmetic result.

You won't come to any harm washing your wound, even the day after your surgery. Just make sure that you pat the wound dry using a soft, clean towel. Keeping the area clean, in fact, helps prevent infection and encourages healing.

During surgery a drainage tube or drain may be placed into the scar over your breast or chest area or into the armpit wound. This may need to stay in for a few days. Some surgeons use drains that connect to a bag that you can empty yourself on a daily basis. If this is the case, keep a record of how much is drained every day. Also, record the color of the fluid, which will slowly change from red, to reddish yellow, to a straw color. We normally remove the drain when less than 25 mL per day drains out over two consecutive days, but please check with your own surgeon. It certainly is a real relief when your drain is out, and you'll feel a lot more comfortable.

On the first day after your surgery, it's good to get up for a walk and sit out of bed. You may need to support your arm when walking or sitting. Practice these exercises:

- Deep breathing and coughing to help open up your air passages after anesthetic
- Bending and straightening elbows, wrists, and fingers
- Bending your ankles and knees to keep your circulation moving
- Squeezing your shoulder blades together.

The most important thing to remember is to try not to stress too much; most problems arising after breast surgery are not emergencies, and they can be managed by you or your family doctor.

Pain

It is not uncommon to have some pain after breast surgery, and usually the recommended dosage of acetaminophen/paracetemol (usually branded as Tylenol/Panadol), with or without codeine, is all that you need. If you're experiencing severe pain, then there may be something wrong, such as a collection of normal tissue fluid that causes pressure but is not dangerous. Or, rarely, there may be a collection of pus (an abscess), which is more serious and requires urgent drainage and antibiotics.

Bruising

Bruising occurs in about one in ten patients and may be more common if you're taking a blood-thinning agent. Try not to take any aspirin before your operation. I have now seen two patients who had a lot of bruising, and we discovered that they drank large amounts of green tea. The concern is the high vitamin K content of green tea leaves, which in excessive amounts could potentially interfere with clotting mechanisms, and therefore cause bleeding or bruising. Most bruising settles down within a two- to four-week period.

Wound swelling

It's not uncommon to get some puffiness or firmness around the scar, and occasionally, some fluid may come out of the scar. Again, don't worry too much, but do check with your doctor.

Seroma

This is a collection of fluid, which normally occurs under the scar in the armpit region but can also occur under the scar of your breast, or even under a mastectomy scar if your breast was removed. This is normal fluid in your body that has leaked a little bit because of surgery. This can cause a swelling under your armpit (like a golf or tennis ball) that will need to be drained by your surgeon using a needle and syringe or by a radiologist under ultrasound control. A seroma nearly always settles down without further surgery.

Numbness

This is not uncommon and usually settles down a lot, particularly three months after surgery. It is most common in the upper and inner part of your arm after an axillary clearance but uncommon after a sentinel node biopsy. What you are left with at 12 months is generally what you can expect for the rest of your life.

Uncommon side effects after surgery

Wound Infection

Occasionally, more difficult complications can occur after surgery, such as a wound infection. When this occurs, the wound may become more painful, red, and hot. If the infection gets into the bloodstream, you may become quite ill and run a fever. If you experience these symptoms, it's important to see your doctor immediately and get some antibiotics. While wound infection happens occasionally, it is very uncommon to get a more serious boil or abscess.

Cording

Some women have pain, tightness, and a fibrous band that feels like a tight cord running from their armpit to the back of the hand. This is called **cording**. It is thought to be due to hardened lymph vessels. Sometimes it can make it difficult to move the arm. Physiotherapy can help, and sometimes antibiotics are given. I find that regular vitamin E massage of the inner arm can be helpful to ease your symptoms. The pain usually gets better gradually over a few months, but can sometimes come back.

Wound problems

You sometimes find you are left with a fatty lump at the outer edge of the scar under your armpit. This lumpy area usually settles over a period of time. Occasionally this extra tissue (called a "dog ear") may also need to be trimmed at a later date.

Wound breakdown, is uncommon, and means that the scar does not look clean, may be red and swollen, and can come apart, which can delay the healing process from a few days to up to about three weeks. More often than not, it's because the blood supply to a small area of skin has been compromised and the wound doesn't heal properly in that area. The body heals this area by forming a scab which eventually falls off. Very rarely, this area may need to be removed by a small operation. It may be more frequent in people who smoke, and apart from an increased chance of chest problems if you smoke, this is another reason why it's a good idea to quit before your surgery.

Once your wound is healed, we advise our patients to massage their scar and surrounding skin with Bio-Oil® in a circular motion, twice a day, for a minimum period of three months. This is used to help improve the appearance of your scar.

When to call your doctor

Call your doctor or breast care nurse immediately if you have:

- A temperature over 38°C or 100.4°F
- Signs of infection such as redness, pain, or swelling
- Signs of an extensive bruise ("hematoma")
- Chest pain and shortness of breath, which may indicate a heart attack or a blood clot in the calf travelling to the chest.

The most important thing is to try not to stress too much; most problems that arise after breast surgery are not emergencies, and they can be managed by you or your family doctor.

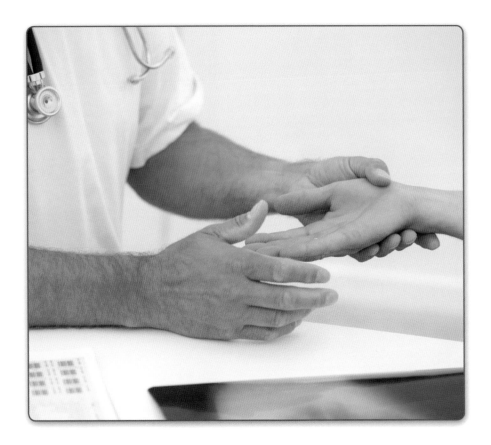

CONTROL POINT #9 – HOW DO I DEAL WITH ANY POSSIBLE COMPLICATIONS?

WARNING

If you have a temperature over 38°C or 100.4°F or any signs of infection such as redness, pain, or swelling, see your doctor immediately for antibiotics.

TIP

On the first day after your surgery, it's good to get up for a walk and sit out of bed. You may need to support your arm when walking or sitting.

REMEMBER

The most important thing is to try not to stress too much; most problems that arise after breast surgery are not emergencies, and they can be managed by you or your family doctor.

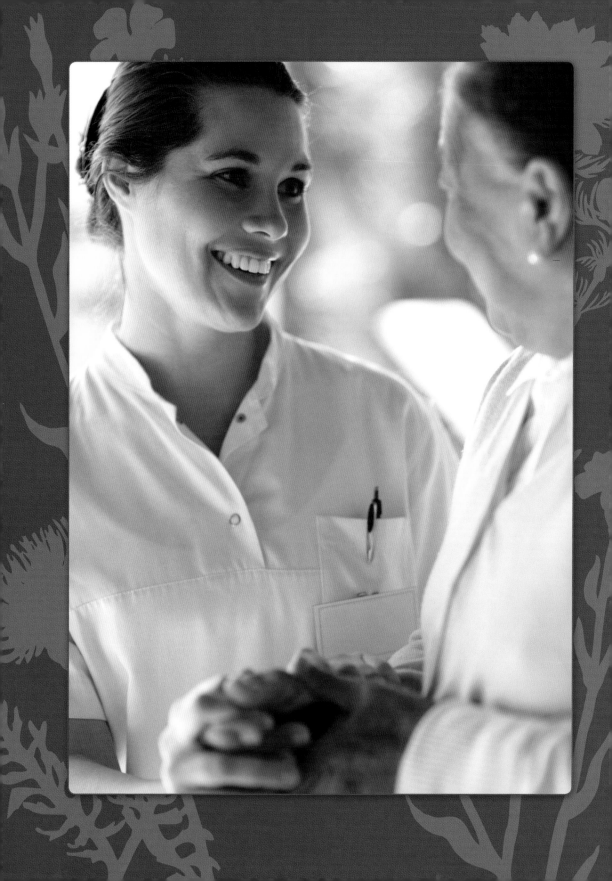

Control Point 10

Do I Need More Surgery?

Control Point #10

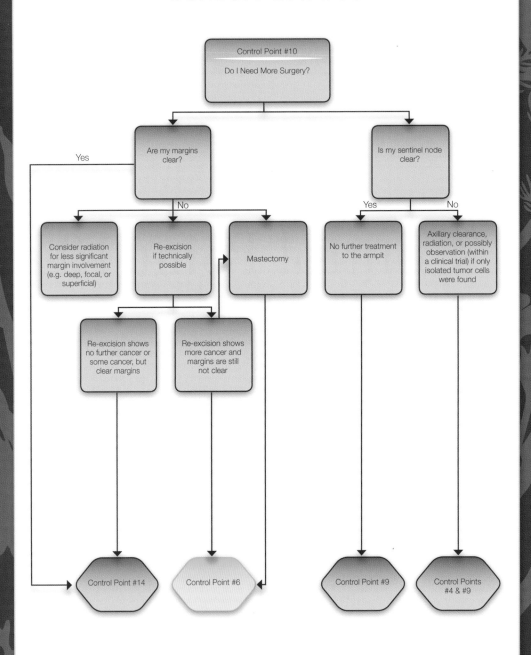

Control Point #10

Do I Need More Surgery?

Are my margins clear?

Is my sentinel node clear?

Yes

No

Yes

No

Consider radiation for less significant margin involvement (e.g. deep, focal, or superficial)

Re-excision if technically possible

Mastectomy

No further treatment to the armpit

Axillary clearance, radiation, or possibly observation (within a clinical trial) if only isolated tumor cells were found

Re-excision shows no further cancer or some cancer, but clear margins

Re-excision shows more cancer and margins are still not clear

Control Point #14

Control Point #6

Control Point #9

Control Points #4 & #9

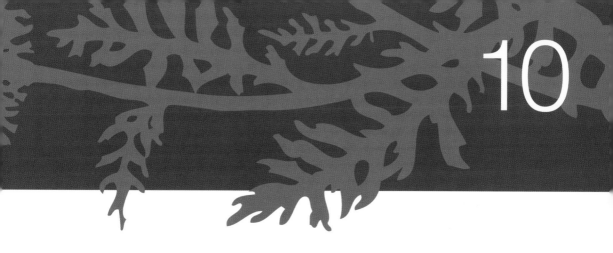

Do I Need More Surgery?

The next important question is, "Do I need any more surgery?" There are two key aspects right now to consider following surgery to your breast and axilla (Figures 63 to 65). It is a particularly stressful time when you need to go back to your doctor's office to be given your results. Make sure you take a support person with you at this very important visit (Figure 66).

Are my margins clear?

During breast conservation surgery, the surgeon often removes a piece of tissue the size of a golf ball, or even larger. The specimen is then labeled by the surgeon using either sutures or inks to tell the pathologist the orientation of the specimen within the breast. This is important for the pathologist to work out what is going on in the margin, or edge, of the specimen. The margin is the distance between your invasive cancer or any pre-cancer (DCIS) and the edge of the tissue that has been removed. If you have had a lumpectomy, then it is important that you have a clear margin, but there's a lot of debate about what a clear margin actually is. In our Institute, we accept margins as small as 0.5 mm, as long as there are no other factors that may result in a higher chance of cancer coming back.

Research from Harvard University examined the distance between the surgical cut and the tumor and the risk of cancer coming back in the breast after surgery and radiation. Recurrence rates in the breast were virtually the same statistically for patients in all categories, including patients who had very close margins, as they were for patients who had a re-excision (a second lumpectomy in the same spot) where no cancer was found at all.

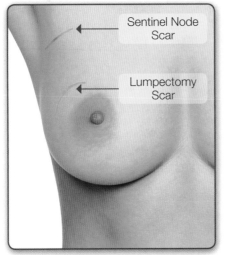

Sentinel Node Scar

Lumpectomy Scar

Figure 63: After surgery, we need to look at what we found in the breast (particularly the margins) and see whether or not the cancer has spread to the armpit (simulated scars are shown).

Table 3 shows these important results (Park 2000). I will go into factors that predict for a higher chance of cancer coming back later.

At this stage, I would like to say that if your margins are clear (even by less than 1 mm) and there are no other abnormal findings (such as an "**extensive intraductal component**" or marked "**lymphatic vessel invasion**"), then you probably don't need more surgery.

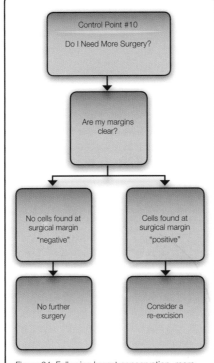

Figure 64: Following breast conservation, more surgery may be required at the site of a positive margin.

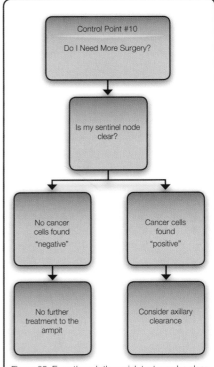

Figure 65: Even though the quick test may be clear, the final, more accurate testing may show that cancer has spread to the glands, and a second operation may be required to remove the remainder of the glands.

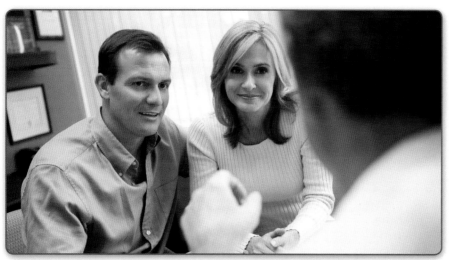

Figure 66: Take a support person with you when you go to see the surgeon for your results.

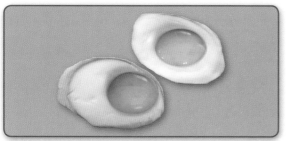

Figure 67: This is an example of a clear, or negative, margin on the top right and a close margin on the bottom left.

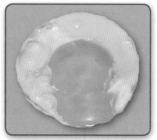

Figure 68: Egg yolk extending to the edge of the white is like a positive margin.

Closest Margin Distance	Number of Patients	Recurrence in the Breast
0.1 – 1.0 mm	94	7%
1.1 – 2.0 mm	33	6%
2.1 – 5.0 mm	47	4%
> 5.0 mm (including no cancer found after a re-excision)	126	9%
Not known	41	7%

Table 3: Chance of a recurrence in the breast after breast conservation with lumpectomy and radiation therapy, based on depth of margin (with permission from the American Society of Clinical Oncology)

Do I Need More Surgery? 161

If cancer is touching the edge of the surgical cut, this is known as a "positive" or "dirty" margin. In figures 67 to 68, I have used a fried egg to clarify what I mean by a clear or "negative" and a close or "positive" margin. The egg yolk represents the cancer, and the egg white the margin of normal breast tissue around the cancer. If you have a positive margin, shown in Figure 68 as the yolk touching the outer edge of the egg white, then you may need an extra "shave" of tissue removed in the area where the margin was positive. Sometimes a mastectomy may be required. In some circumstances, when an extra margin cannot be obtained with more surgery or when the margin involvement is minimal or "focal," radiotherapy can also be given.

Is my sentinel node biopsy clear?

The next decision that needs to be made is whether or not you require more surgery for the lymph glands under your armpit. You may recall from earlier that the sentinel node is thought to be the first draining lymph node that acts as a filter trap for any cancer cells that may have spread from the cancer in your breast, and that the surgeon usually does a quick test on your sentinel node while you're anesthetized.

Unfortunately, the quick test is only about 50 percent accurate, and even after a negative quick test, some patients do receive the disappointing news that the final sentinel node test shows some cancer cells. This is called a "positive sentinel node" (Figure 65). In this situation, the surgeon may book you in for a full axillary clearance (where the surgeon goes back and takes out the rest of your lymph glands in your armpit) in the next week or so, or he or she may make a decision not to put you through any more surgery.

The sentinel node testing protocol by the examining pathologist is now so thorough that we often detect cancer cells that we would not have known existed perhaps five or ten years ago. So please don't get too concerned if your sentinel node is involved. It may indeed be the only node involved, or if it only shows a "touch of cancer" (or, to use the medical word, a micro-metastasis or isolated tumor cells (ITCs), then the chances of other lymph glands being involved may be very low.

There are ongoing clinical trials testing whether it's safe to simply observe the armpit instead of having more surgery if only an ITC or a micro-metastasis is found. If a sentinel node is definitely involved, and particularly if a pathologist can see the cancer cells without the assistance of immuno-histochemical stains, then there's about a 40 percent chance that other lymph glands are involved. It's important in this case to organize more surgery or sometimes radiation therapy.

The Memorial Sloan-Kettering Cancer Center's website provides a calculator that works out the probability of additional lymph glands being involved if the sentinel node is involved.

Click the "Calculate Risk" button after you click the link below:

www.mskcc.org/mskcc/applications/nomograms_v2/BreastNonSLN.aspx

The prospect of facing more surgery is very frustrating and may feel like another hill you have to climb, but hang in there. The good news is that your treatment team has found the exact location of the cancer cells and will now tailor the best treatment plan for your particular circumstances.

CONTROL POINT #10 – DO I NEED MORE SURGERY?

WARNING

If a sentinel node is definitely involved, and particularly if a pathologist can see the cancer cells without the assistance of immuno-histochemical stains, then there's about a four in ten chance that other lymph glands are involved in your armpit.

TIP

After breast conservation, even a close margin of less than 1mm may be safe when you have follow-up radiation therapy.

REMEMBER

The two important parts of your pathology report that determine the need for more surgery are whether or not the margins of excision are clear and whether or not cancer cells are found in your sentinel node.

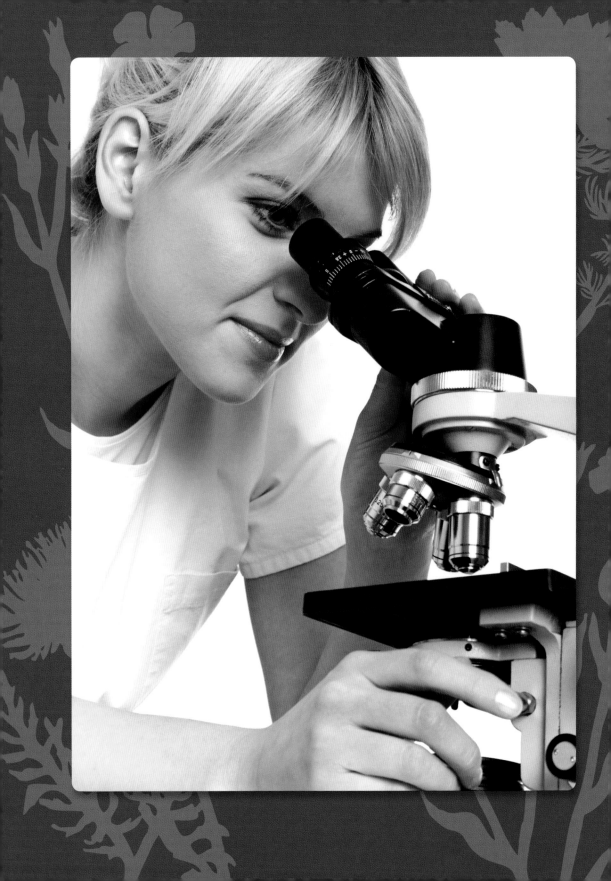

Control Point 11

What Does My Pathology Report Really Mean?

Control Point #11

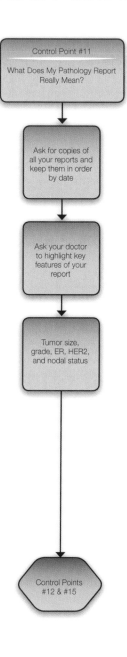

Control Point #11

What Does My Pathology Report
Really Mean?

Ask for copies of
all your reports and
keep them in order
by date

Ask your doctor
to highlight key
features of your
report

Tumor size,
grade, ER, HER2,
and nodal status

Control Points
#12 & #15

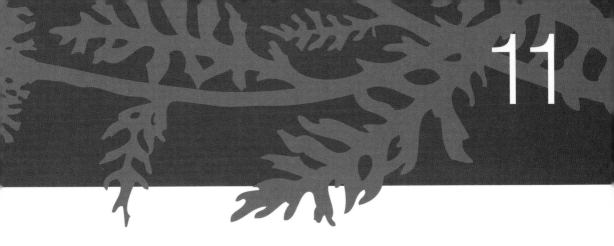

What Does My Pathology Report Really Mean?

The next step is for you and your doctor to understand your pathology report fully. The pathology report can be a bit scary—it's usually in very detailed medical language that may not make sense. Some of my patients get frightened by reading some aspects of the report.

The pathology report looks at your breast cancer (what I called a "weed" in the garden example earlier) in very fine detail. It described not only what the "weed" looks like when you view it with the naked eye (the **macroscopic report**), but also what its real structure looks like under the microscope (the **microscopic report**) (Figure 69). The pathologist works out whether it's a weed that can spread its seed to other parts of the garden, or one that starts and finishes in the same patch of garden. On the next few pages, I list what needs to be recorded in a good "structured" report. This is essentially a checklist of what the pathologist should document in the report and is now included in many international guidelines.

Unfortunately, many pathologists still use a "paraphrased" report, which is a long narrative. I find these quite difficult to read, and sometimes important information is not clearly stated. The structured report, on the other hand, allows the oncologist to find the important elements (or factors) in your pathology quickly, and it also highlights the important aspects of the report to you.

Tables 7, on page 180, show the risks of a recurrence in the breast after breast conservation, or on the chest wall or lymph glands above the breastbone after a mastectomy ("**local recurrence**"), or in other parts of the body (**metastatic disease**)

associated with various pathologic features that may be present in your cancer. Remember that many cancers may have a mixture of "good" and "not so good" features. Refer to this table if something is not clear in your pathology report.

You see, not all factors are "equal." Some factors may predict a higher chance of the cancer coming back somewhere else, and therefore indicate that treatment may be required for the rest of the body. Other factors may predict a higher chance of cancer coming back in the breast, but not necessarily elsewhere in the body.

Some factors may indicate that the cancer is a type of "weed" that can blow in the wind and drop its seeds elsewhere in the garden. If that's the case, then we really need to have a good strong think about treatments that go to all parts of the body, such as chemotherapy or hormonal treatment. If a factor predicts for a local recurrence (where the cancer could come back in the same place or region of the breast), then you may need more treatment, such as a mastectomy or further surgery, such as an "extra shave"(re-excision).

Do remember, however, that the pathology report is only an indication. There is always hope and it's important for you to do what you can to take back control. Understand your report, but don't get too overwhelmed if there are a few "negative" findings. Usually, there are "positive" findings as well.

The real point is that nobody can predict their future. Often, a breast cancer diagnosis has a better prognosis than a heart attack or even diabetes. At other times, yes, breast cancer can come back, but even in situations where the disease looks advanced, I have known many women who were still alive 20 or even 30 years later.

The pathology report is complicated. Ask for a photocopy of it. It is your breast and your breast tumor, and you really need to know what's going on. Be polite but firm.

There are two parts to the pathology report. As mentioned, the first section is called the macroscopic report and the second section is called the microscopic report. Further tests are conducted in the pathology lab on your breast cancer to work out whether it is likely to respond to hormonal treatments or Herceptin. These extra tests take longer than the routine testing and often two or three "amended" or "updated" reports are issued after your original report.

Understanding the macroscopic report

The macroscopic report addresses what can be seen with the naked eye. It's not usually done by the specialist pathologist, but perhaps by an assistant, such as a resident in training. Parts of it may be documented by a technician.

The macroscopic report includes:

- The type of specimen (a breast conservation specimen or a mastectomy specimen)

- If there are any scars on the skin or if the nipple is present

- The dimensions (and sometimes the weight) of the excised specimen

- The dimensions of the macroscopic tumor. In other words, if they can see an abnormality that looks like a cancer, they may measure it at this point. This is usually measured in millimeters or centimeters, but sometime inches.

- The distance between the tumor and the cut edge of the specimen (the margin)

- The presence of any other abnormalities, such as a second unsuspected or previously discovered cancer

- An indication of which parts or "sections" of the specimen (called "blocks") have been sampled

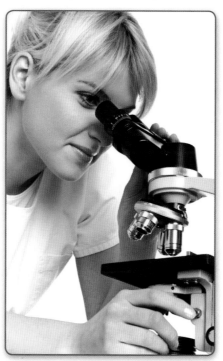

Figure 69: It can take more than a week for a final pathology report; it can be a long wait. A pathologist uses a microscope to check lots and lots of slides of your tumor.

These are the six most important aspects, particularly if breast conservation was done. I use these six aspects to work out how much normal tissue the surgeon has removed compared to the size of the breast tumor, and to calculate how close the cancer is to the edge of the specimen. The two most important aspects are how big the cancer is, and if it's been removed.

Understanding the microscopic report

The section below is quite detailed and you may want to skip part or all of it. This is what I look for in the microscopic report:

Type of procedure

Confirm that breast conservation or mastectomy was done (this is sometimes only recorded at the top of the report in the macroscopic section).

Tumor site or location

It's important to correlate what is seen on the pathology report with what was seen on the pre-operative mammogram or ultrasound and with where you felt a breast lump if one was present. Some pathologists go to the trouble of documenting the location of the tumor, but usually in terms of a quadrant (or a quarter of the breast). The most common location is the upper outer quadrant, which is the quarter toward the armpit, as shown earlier in Figure 26.

Tumor type

This is a summary of the different types of cancers mentioned above. The most common type of cancers are invasive ductal carcinoma and then invasive lobular carcinoma (Figures 9 and 10). What I look for here are special types of tumors, such as tubular or mucinous carcinomas which tend to have a better prognosis (Figures 11 and 12).

Pathologic size of the tumor

Most pathologists measure a tumor in three dimensions. For example, a tumor might be 20 x 10 x 10 mm. Sometimes a second area of cancer or focus is mentioned, and in a good report, the distance between the two "foci" or spots of cancer is usually documented (as in Figures 27 and 28).

It's important to be sure that only the invasive tumor size is measured. Make sure that you or your doctors do not add the size of the invasive carcinoma to the size of the pre-cancer, because the prognosis is determined by the size of the invasive cancer. The extent of the pre-invasive area doesn't really matter all that much for prognosis but may determine the need for further surgery or radiotherapy.

We generally work out how advanced a cancer in the breast is using an international convention of stages, known as tumor stages, specifically for the tumor ("T") in your breast (Table 4).

Tumor Stage	Diameter of the Tumor or Features
T1	0–20 mm
T1a	0–5 mm
T1b	> 5–10 mm
T1c	> 10–20 mm
T2	> 20–50 mm
T3	> 50 mm
T4	Tumor involving the skin or chest wall

Table 4: Defining the tumor (or "T") stage means categorizing the size of the cancer in your breast

Histologic grade

The histologic grade of the cancer is determined by three components. This was originally documented by two famous pathologists named Bloom and Richardson.

They worked out that three sub-components can add up to a score from 1 to 9 that may determine prognosis. The three components of grade are:

- **Nuclear grade:** This is how abnormal the nucleus (or control center) of the cancer cell looks. This is scored in a range from 1 to 3. For the **nuclear grade**, the pathologist looks at the size of the nucleus, its shape, and its staining intensity, which helps to determine how much DNA content it has and whether it's highly abnormal (score 3) or closer to a normal cell (score 1).

- **Tubule formation:** The normal breast has tubules, which are the ducts that carry milk from the lobules (or leaves) to the nipple (Figure 5). The more tubules your cancer has, the more it's like a normal breast, and therefore the lower its grade. Once again, this is scored 1, 2, or 3. With higher-grade cancers, i.e. a score of 3, there are only a few or no tubules. At the lower end of the spectrum, the tumor may be an "infiltrating tubular" cancer that consists mainly of tubules. Such a tumor has a score of 1 and is more like normal breast tissue, as shown in Figure 11.

- **Mitotic rate:** This is the number of cells that seem to be dividing at a given time. **Mitosis** is where one cell divides into two cells and it is basically how a cancer keeps growing. Cells undergoing mitosis are arrowed in Figure 70. The pathologist normally counts the number of cells dividing per ten high-power fields. (This refers to the setting on the microscope viewer.) An example of the Bloom–Richardson score (or grade) is shown in Table 5.

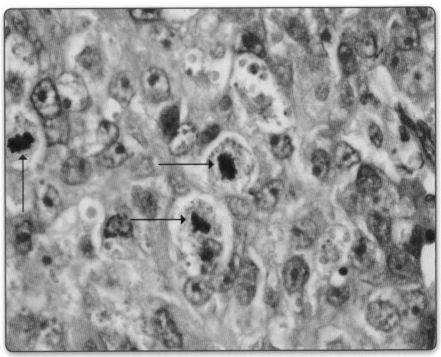

Figure 70: Infiltrating (invasive) duct carcinoma cells (arrowed) undergoing division (or "mitosis").

Bloom–Richardson Score	1	2	3
Tubule Formation	X		
Nuclear Grade		X	
Mitotic Rate		X	

Table 5: Components of the Bloom–Richardson histological score for a patient with a grade 1 tumor

Total Bloom–Richardson Score	3-5	6-7	8-9
Histologic Grade	1 (low)	2 (intermediate)	3 (high)

Table 6: Calculating the histologic grade of a tumor

This patient has a score of 1 + 2 + 2 = 5. You can see in Table 6 that a score of 5 is a "low-grade" or "grade 1" tumor.

The grade of a cancer is one of the most important factors in determining whether chemotherapy is required. Even small grade 3 tumors (particularly those measuring over 10 mm), with no spread to the lymph glands, are probably best

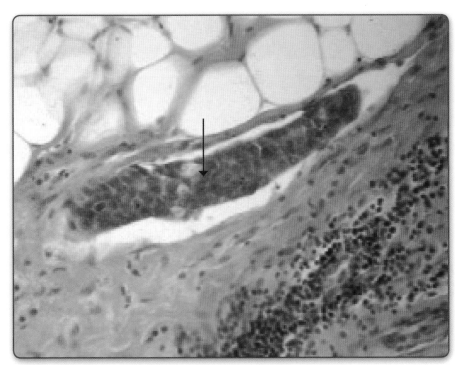

Figure 71: The presence of cancer cells in a lymphatic channel (arrowed) is called lymphatic vessel invasion (LVI).

treated with chemotherapy in addition to surgery and/or radiation therapy.

The pathologist has to make various judgments to work out the components of grade, so it can be a little subjective at times. Some grade 2 tumors may behave more like grade 1 tumors and others more like grade 3 tumors. Don't get too anxious about grade, as we now have very effective treatments for tumors of all grades and it's only one of many factors that we look at to work out prognosis and treatment.

Margins of resection

This is quite a controversial area. No pathologist can really hold their hand on their heart and say that a margin is truly negative or positive. The first problem is that the pathologist can only report on what's been removed. An International Consensus Conference was convened in Milan, Italy, in 2005, with a group of experts in breast cancer and breast conservation representing each of the disciplines involved in the care of these patients. Margins were one of the areas where consensus was not reached (Schwartz 2006). The panelists agreed to disagree about the width of the margins required after breast conservation; they all concurred that there should be no evidence of tumor at the transected edge of the excision (like the yolk and the egg white in Figure 67), and most radiation oncologists were comfortable with a margin of at least 1–2 mm (see also Table 3).

Vascular or lymphatic invasion

Essentially, this is where a pathologist sees cancer in a space that looks like a blood vessel or lymphatic vessel (Figure 71). Vascular invasion of the cancer can be misleading; some pathologists call it lymphovascular invasion, as it's often very difficult for the pathologist to determine whether it's in the lymph or a blood vessel.

The problem with **lymphovascular invasion** is that sometimes it can be an artifact (a false reading or impression) because of some shrinkage of the specimen when it's being processed by the pathologist. On the other hand, it may be a sign that the cancer is spreading into the small lymphatic vessels or blood vessels, and some studies have found this to predict for a slightly higher chance of the cancer coming back somewhere else in the body. A few studies have also found that when lymphovascular invasion (or "LVI"), is extensive, it may also be a risk factor for a recurrence on the chest wall or in the breast.

When it's just present "focally," or in just one spot, I don't worry too much about it and don't see it as a strong reason to give radiation therapy after a mastectomy. If the pathologist says it's extensive throughout the cut specimen and at the margin, then it's best to play it safe and consider a re-excision and sometimes post-mastectomy radiation. The presence of LVI has been associated with a higher risk of the cancer spreading to the lymph glands, as shown in Jill's case below.

Number of axillary lymph glands found

This can be quite misleading. Different pathology departments can find different numbers of lymph glands in the same sample, and it may depend on the quality control and the technique used in a particular lab. Sometimes when we find too few lymph glands, we kindly ask the pathologist to check again, and occasionally more lymph glands are found.

Often, residents or technicians "dissect" the axillary specimen looking for these lymph glands, and the number found depends on factors such as the experience of the pathologist, the lab protocols, and the technician's technique. As explained above, it is good practice to find at least ten, and preferably 15, lymph glands in the armpit or axilla. There are usually fewer lymph glands found after chemotherapy.

Jill's Story

Jill was only 31 at the time and was a sonographer (a technician who uses ultrasound) and was just married. She found a lump in her breast, scanned herself, and had a mammogram in the practice where she worked.

The mammogram was clear, and the radiologist thought the lump could be watched, but she insisted on a biopsy.

This came back as atypical, and the surgeon, thinking (or more likely hoping) that it was benign, insisted on taking it out right away under a local anesthetic, which caused some bruising.

The lump came back as a 4 mm, grade 3 cancer with some lymphatic vessel invasion . The surgeon wasn't really keen on taking out the glands under her armpit, but I insisted because of the high grade and vessel invasion. To our surprise, one gland was involved with cancer. This was before the time of sentinel node procedures.

Jill emailed me recently. She is living a full and active life and has had two healthy children since her treatment, now school-aged.

Number of positive axillary lymph glands found

This is the most important prognostic factor. Finding "positive" lymph glands means that cancer cells have moved from "first base" in your breast to "second base" in your armpit. Using my garden example, it's like the weed spreading from the first to the adjacent second garden patch. The pathology report will differentiate between the sentinel and non-sentinel nodes found. Some surgeons remove non-axillary sentinel nodes or lymph glands that are found in locations other than the armpit, such as the internal mammary nodes, or the lymph glands under the breastbone ("infra-clavicular"), and these are also labeled. Women who have no nodes involved have a better prognosis than women with involved nodes.

For convenience, many oncologists group women into several nodal categories:

Node negative: There is no doubt that this is the best situation to be in. We have more confidence that your armpit lymph glands are truly negative if ten or more glands are dissected (Axelsson 2009).

Isolated tumor cells (ITCs): This can be a difficult situation. ITCs are defined as single tumor cells or small cell clusters, not larger than 0.2 mm, that are usually detected only by immuno-histochemical (IHC) or molecular methods. They may also be verified by the naked eye using purple stains (Figures 70 and 71) known as hematoxylin & eosin (H&E) stains. There is a lot of controversy about what to do if a pathologist finds ITCs as part of their workup of the sentinel node.

One of the best review papers about the significance of micro-metastases in lymph glands was published in 2003 by the *European Journal of Cancer*. The European Working Group for Breast Screening Pathology was founded in 1993, and at that time, the group consisted of 30 pathologists from all member states of the European Union (Cserni 2003).

They wisely state that "It is unclear how often these isolated tumor cells reflect metastases capable of further growth and dissemination (spread)." The review examined 13 studies to determine whether ITCs had a negative impact on prognosis. Five of the 13 studies showed that ITCs had a negative impact on prognosis, whereas the majority (eight studies) found no impact on prognosis.

Micro-metastases: These are larger than ITCs but still less than 2 mm. The European Working Group noted that "Micro-metastases are more likely to denote a prognostic disadvantage because of their larger size, although no evidence for this is available." If discovered, micro-metastases are probably best regarded as an indication for systemic adjuvant treatment such as chemotherapy or hormonal treatment.

Non-sentinel node involvement (NSN): Several studies have looked at the probability of cancer going beyond an involved sentinel node. In research in which I have been involved at the Institute, we found that the overall rate of non-sentinel node (NSN) involvement was 40 percent once one sentinel node was found to be involved with cancer. However, the risk is lower if the sentinel node is only slightly involved with ITCs or a micro-metastasis.

The European Working Group estimated that nearly one in five patients (18 percent) with only small deposits in their sentinel node (ITCs or micro-metastases) would have disease in the axilla after a dissection, and probably as low as one in ten (12 percent) if the sentinel node only had disease present that was detectable only by special stains (immuno-histochemistry) and not seen by the naked eye.

Definite nodal involvement: 1–3 positive nodes, 4–9 positive nodes, or 10 or more positive nodes: This involves a simple count by the pathologist of how many lymph glands are involved. The pathologist also records if the cancer has spread outside the outer boundary or capsule of the node. This is called "**extracapsular spread**" or "**extranodal spread**" or extension, and if it's over 4 or 5 mm, it may be an indication for radiation to the axilla after surgery.

Nodes in the internal mammary chain: Depending on local practice, the sentinel node procedure may pick up radioactive uptake in the internal mammary chain, located just on the edge of the breastbone, and which may be removed during your surgery (Figure 35). These lymph glands are more likely to be involved if you are under the age of 40, if you have a bigger cancer (over 50 mm), if your tumor is located in the inner quadrants, or if the lymph glands in the armpit are involved.

There are ongoing trials to see whether or not giving this area radiation may improve prognosis or reduce the chance of a recurrence. Some radiation oncologists do treat this area if they consider the risk to be higher than normal, but the trade-off will involve slightly higher radiation doses to the skin, and possibly an increased dose to the heart.

Nodes in the inter-pectoral region (Rotter's nodes): Occasionally, we find a gland tucked in between the two pectoral muscles (Figure 35). These were first discovered by Rotter in 1896. As many as 50 percent of women have a Rotter's node, and if found, it can contain cancer in one in five cases. Rotter's nodes are more frequently involved if there are many other lymph glands, and involved nodes would be treated by chemotherapy and possibly radiation therapy. Your surgeon would normally take a look between the two muscles when he or she is performing an axillary clearance, and place any abnormal looking tissue in a separate specimen jar for testing. It is very rare for a Rotter's node to be the only site of nodal involvement.

The estrogen receptor

Perhaps as many as 80 percent of women who are older and 50 to 60 percent of women who are younger (under the age of 50) may have an estrogen receptor (ER)-positive tumor. The estrogen receptor is like an antenna on the cell. Many normal parts of the female body need **estrogen**. These include the brain, the breast, the vagina, and the bones. I will talk a lot more about this later in Control Point #16 —Do I Need Hormonal Treatment?

Estrogen receptors look for estrogen, and when they bind with the estrogen, it generates a sequence of chemical changes that activate changes within the cell. The association between **hormone replacement therapy** ("HRT") and an increased risk of breast cancer is thought to be due to HRT "feeding" a pre-existent cancer cell with estrogen, which can make it grow. It's a bit like giving fertilizer to a weed.

Theoretically, ER-positive cells may grow with estrogen produced by your body. Estrogen can be produced even after menopause. In younger women, it is produced by the ovaries and in muscle, fat, and adrenal glands (which produce androgens and enzymes that control your blood pressure and are located above the kidneys).

The more like a normal breast cell your cancer is, the more likely that the cancer cell will have retained its estrogen receptors. These cancers tend to be of lower grade and tend to have a better prognosis. The other advantage of ER-positive tumors is that we have more options for treatment. ER-positive tumors can be treated with adjuvant (additional) hormonal treatments such as **tamoxifen** or **aromatase inhibitors**. Adjuvant treatment is generally given after surgery and could be radiation, chemotherapy, or hormonal treatment. Treatment given before surgery is called **neo-adjuvant treatment**.

Having an ER-positive tumor does not necessarily mean that you won't need chemotherapy, but it may mean that hormonal treatment will be significantly more beneficial or as good as chemotherapy. Further, some patients with smaller tumors (under 10–20 mm), or perhaps patients who are older, may just need hormonal treatment alone.

Progesterone receptors (PRs) are a similar type of receptor and are thought to be functional only when an estrogen receptor is present. We don't fully understand how the two interact, but there is some evidence that some patients who are PR-positive may respond better to aromatase inhibitors than to drugs like tamoxifen—however we're not entirely sure about this.

The HER2 receptor

The HER2 receptor is present in all cells in our body. The problem is that in one in five patients with breast cancer, part of the HER2 receptor has gone a little bit crazy and becomes "over-expressed." The HER2 receptor controls cell growth, and patients with HER2-positive tumors may have cancers that are more aggressive and divide more rapidly.

There are two different ways that we measure the HER2 receptor. The quick test is performed with immuno-histochemistry and is the most commonly used test. It's measured by a scoring system of 1, 2, or 3.

The other type of testing is called an **ISH (in-situ hybridization)** test, which is more accurate but takes a week or two for the result. Don't get too worried by the techniques (including FISH, CISH or SISH tests) that are used, before we recommend Herceptin, a drug that binds and blocks the HER2 receptor (see Control Point #19—Do I Need Herceptin (Trastuzumab)?).

There isn't one ideal test for working out prognosis. We certainly don't know a lot about what to do with patients with very small cancers that have lots of good features, but one or two not so good features (such as grade 3 or HER2 positivity). Currently, we tend to recommend some chemotherapy in these patients, but more research is going on right now to determine whether all patients who are HER2 positive need to be treated with drugs such as Herceptin.

Triple-negative breast cancer

This is a relatively new term to describe a breast cancer that is HER2-negative, ER-negative, and PR-negative. Young African–American women have a higher incidence of triple-negative disease than white women, as do women with the breast cancer gene. These tumors do not respond to anti-hormonal treatments, but standard chemotherapy can still work. A lot of research is being done on this group of tumors to improve their prognosis and to work out which chemotherapy agents work better against them.

Factor	Predictor of Recurrence in the Breast after Breast Conservation	Predictor of Recurrence on the Chest Wall or Lymph Glands above the Collarbone after a Mastectomy	Predictor of Disease Coming Back in Another Part of the Body (Metastatic Disease)
Very Young Age (< 35 years at diagnosis)	Yes	Yes; at least two studies have found this, but it's not a major factor on its own and not an indicator for chest wall radiation	Yes, but depends a lot on the number of lymph glands involved, as well
Tumor Size	Not a major factor	Yes, particularly if the tumor measures over 50 mm	Increasing tumor size is associated with increased risk of disease elsewhere in the body
Histologic Grade	Not a major factor on its own	Not a major factor on its own	Grade 3 tumors have a higher risk, even when glands are clear
Tumor Type	Some but not all studies have found a slightly higher chance with infiltrating lobular cancers	Some but not all studies have found a slightly higher chance with infiltrating lobular cancers	No
Lymphatic Vessel Invasion	If extensive, this may predict a higher chance, particularly if there are other factors present (such as EIC) or you are very young	Yes, if extensive. I don't normally consider it to be that important if it's the only factor and only in one spot (focal) rather than extensive	Some studies have found this to be an additional risk factor for metastatic disease
Extensive Intraductal Component (EIC)	No, if the margins of excision are clear	No	No
Positive Lymph Nodes	No	Yes, particularly if there are four or more involved nodes	The more nodes that are involved, the higher the chance of the cancer spreading to another part of the body
Estrogen Receptor (ER)-positive	No	No	Lower if ER-positive and higher if ER-negative
HER2-positive	Not much research yet, but theoretically yes	Not much research yet, but theoretically yes	Yes, HER2-positive cancers have a higher chance of spreading to other parts of the body

Table 7: How factors present in your cancer predict for a future problem in the same breast, the chest wall after a mastectomy, or in other parts of the body

Extensive intraductal component ("EIC")

The Harvard Group found that the presence of a lot of pre-cancer or DCIS inside and surrounding the invasive cancer, which they called an extensive intraductal component or "EIC," was associated with a higher risk of recurrence if breast conservation was done. My PhD thesis was on this factor, and ultimately, we showed that if we could get around this extensive intraductal component with a clear margin, then the risks of breast cancer coming back were within normal limits (Boyages 1990).

Women with EIC had a recurrence rate of about 30 percent in five years, compared to 5 percent of the women who did not have EIC. Today, many other studies have also found that as long as you have a clear margin, then there is no need to worry about having an EIC in your cancer.

However, for women who are very young (34 years of age or under), the presence of EIC and other factors such as extensive lymphatic vessel invasion need to be taken into account, as the two factors together are associated with quite a high rate of local recurrence.

Tables 7 summarizes how the microscopic features of your tumor may impact on the cancer coming back or on your treatment.

CONTROL POINT #11 – WHAT DOES MY PATHOLOGY REPORT REALLY MEAN?

WARNING The pathology report can be a bit scary. It's usually in very detailed medical language that may not make sense. Ask for a copy and ask your doctors to explain and highlight the key points.

TIP Nobody can predict their future. Sometimes a breast cancer diagnosis has a better prognosis than a heart attack or diabetes. Even in situations where the disease looks advanced, many women are still alive 20 or even 30 years later.

REMEMBER There is always hope and it's important for you to do what you can to take control. Understand your pathology report, but don't get too overwhelmed if there are a few negative findings. Usually, there are positive findings as well.

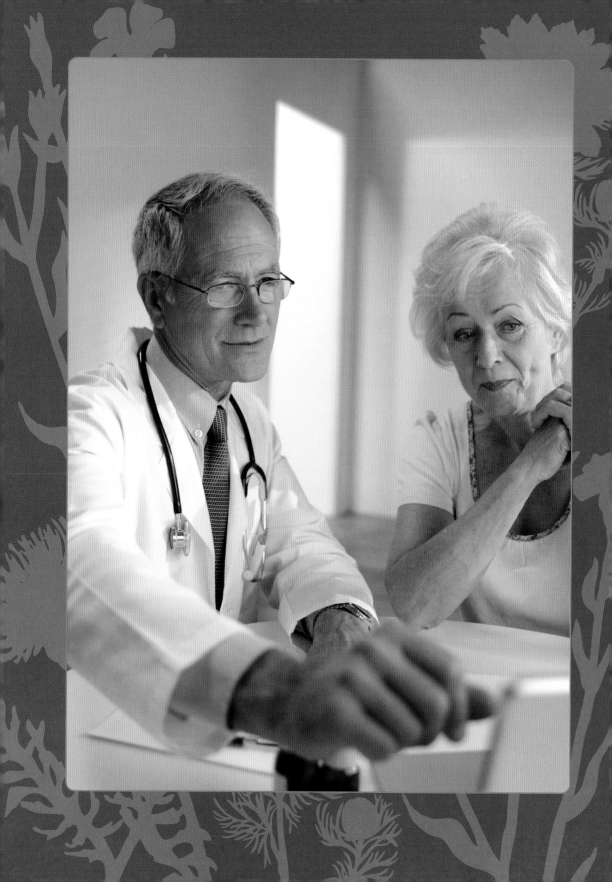

Control Point 12

What Is My Prognosis?

Control Point #12

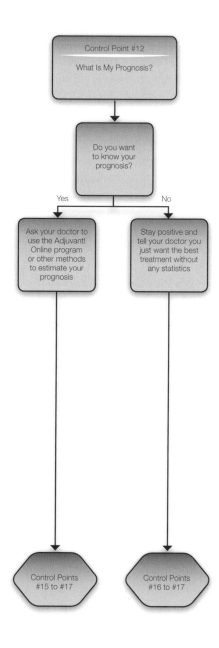

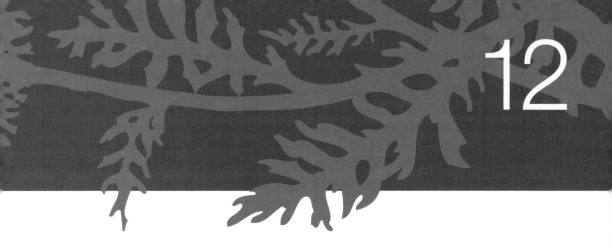

What Is My Prognosis?

Prognosis can be difficult to estimate

This is a very common question that isn't always easy to answer. There are many factors involved in working out prognosis. It's important to stay positive and focused. Remember that a prognosis is just a figure at the point at which you receive it. For most people, the prognosis gets better with time.

Sometimes we use a five-year figure because we know that if cancer comes back, most of the time it comes back within five years. If the cancer has not come back within five years, then the chance of it coming back within ten years is quite low, and if it does not come back within ten years, then you have an almost normal life expectancy.

It's a bit like buying a secondhand car. You don't really know how long it's going to last, but if it lasts year after year without breaking down, then the car starts to look more and more reliable to make that long trip.

Working out a prognosis can be difficult. There's a very good calculator available online at www.adjuvantonline.com, but it's restricted to doctors, so you will need to ask yours to use it for you.

The illustration below shows the type of output that the Adjuvant! Online calculator gives the doctor, who can then print it out for you (Figure 72). From there, the doctor can add in types of treatments, including tamoxifen, aromatase inhibitors, or different types of chemotherapies, to work out your prognosis. Not all people need chemotherapy or hormonal treatment.

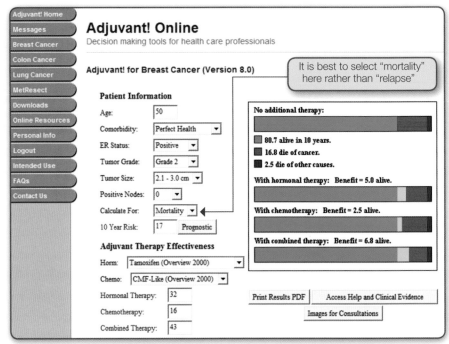

Figure 72: Sample of Adjuvant! Online output showing the "Mortality" setting instead of "Relapse."

Traditional methods of estimating your prognosis

In general, the smaller the cancer in your breast and the fewer the number of lymph glands containing cancer in your armpit, the better your prognosis. Table 8 below shows the ten-year survival rates for someone aged 50 with a grade 2, estrogen receptor-positive (ER-positive) tumor. It shows the survival benefit if treated with hormonal treatment and "second generation" chemotherapy (see Control Point 17) for various combinations of tumor size and involved lymph glands derived from the Adjuvant! Online calculator.

What is pretty clear is that for most situations, the ten-year prognosis is 75 percent or over particularly if the cancer has not spread to more than three glands in the armpit, which is better than a lot of other possible diseases. When the tumor has not spread to the lymph glands, the prognosis is over 85 percent. Pay close attention to your own situation, because the prognosis is slightly better if you have a grade 1 tumor and slightly worse for a grade 3 or an estrogen receptor–negative (ER-negative) tumor.

Ask your oncologist to give you the printout from Adjuvant! Online using the "Calculate for 'Mortality'" setting (see arrow in Figure 72 above). The program's inventor, Dr. Peter Ravdin, clearly states in the fine print to use mortality calculations, since relapse calculations can overestimate the risk of cancer recurrence in the future.

		Number of Involved Lymph Glands in your Armpit			
		0	1–3	4–9	>9
Tumor Size (mm)	1–10	98.5%	92.0%	83.0%	69.0%
	11–20	96.0%	92.0%	83.0%	69.0%
	21–30	91.5%	82.0%	76.0%	62.0%
	31–50	88.0%	82.0%	76.0%	62.0%
	>50	86.0%	75.0%	67.0%	51.0%

Table 8: Ten year survival rates for a 50-year-old woman with a grade 2 hormone receptor positive breast cancer treated with chemotherapy and hormonal treatment

Relapse calculations include all sorts of "events" that can happen, including getting a cancer in the other breast or dying of something else such as old age. Using relapse calculations tends to lead to an overestimation of the benefit of chemotherapy or hormonal treatment.

In the UK and parts of Europe, many doctors use an index developed in Nottingham (Galea 1992). The "NPI," or Nottingham Prognostic Index, is currently calculated using the following factors:

- The size of the cancer
- Whether or not the cancer has spread to the lymph glands under the arm (and if so, how many nodes are affected)
- The grade of the cancer.

The formula is:

NPI = (0.2 x tumor diameter in centimeters) + lymph gland stage + tumor grade

The lymph gland stage is either 1 (if there are no nodes affected), 2 (if one to three glands are affected), or 3 (if four or more glands are affected). Similarly, the tumor grade is scored as 1 to 3 as defined in Control Point #11. Applying the formula gives scores that fall into three bands:

- A score of less than 3.4 suggests a good outcome with a high chance of survival
- A score of between 3.4 to 5.4 is an intermediate level with a moderate chance of survival
- A score of more than 5.4 suggests a smaller likelihood of survival.

It has been validated in more recent patient groups around the world, but although the NPI is a useful guide, like all indices or measures it is not a guarantee of what will happen to you.

Your doctor will look at other factors such as the absolute number of involved lymph glands in the axilla, HER2 and estrogen status of your tumor, whether your tumor is a special type (like tubular or mucinous), and its mitotic rate before making final decisions about your treatment.

Nevertheless, the NPI is very useful as a quick, "back of the envelope" way of working out a category of prognosis without using a computer (like Adjuvant! Online) or more expensive tests described below.

New methods of estimating your prognosis

Researchers have in recent years classified breast cancer into five different sub-types according to its "genetic profile" or "signature." To date, the various sub-types have not been that helpful in making treatment decisions over and above the standard factors that influence prognosis, such as tumor size, grade, nodal status, and so on, but I will discuss them here because you may encounter these terms during your treatment journey.

These genetic profiles include two sub-groups that are ER-positive, called "luminal A" and "luminal B," and three sub-groups that are ER-negative, called "normal breast-like," "HER2-positive," and "basal-like" (or "triple negative").

Other investigators have focused on a limited number of genes to work out how combinations of these genes can classify women with breast cancer into better or worse prognosis groups to help with the choice of having chemotherapy.

The Oncotype DX test is a commercially available diagnostic genetic test that can predict breast cancer recurrence and the likelihood of chemotherapy working if you have a small ER-positive breast cancer which has not spread to the lymph glands and will be treated with tamoxifen. It examines 21 different genes.

Oncotype DX can be performed in the US on paraffin-embedded tissue. Collecting tissue samples in this manner is standard practice on all surgical cases, making this gene assay more readily available. The test did cost a few thousand dollars last time I inquired, so you need to decide if it's worthwhile for you. Information from the manufacturer, Genomic Health, is available from their website: www.oncotypedx.com.

Other genetic tests known as microarrays are also commercially available. MammaPrint® is a gene-expression profiling test that predicts the risk of metastasis in breast cancer patients by analyzing 70 different genes. It's based on groundbreaking research performed at the Netherlands Cancer Institute and the Antoni Van Leeuwenhoek Hospital in Amsterdam. One practical problem is that it requires fresh tissue and cannot be performed on formalin-fixed, paraffin-embedded tumor tissue, as the OncoDX test can. More information is available from the following web site: www.agendia.com/

Another group in Europe has developed the "Genomic Grade Index," also called MapQuant Dx™, and more information about it is available at www.ipsogen.com. This test also requires fresh tissue for testing and examines 97 different genes.

My overall view is that these tests are useful for only a small number of women and have not become a part of routine clinical care.

CONTROL POINT #12 – WHAT IS MY PROGNOSIS?

WARNING Ask your oncologist to use the Adjuvant! Online program to calculate your prognosis using the "Mortality" setting, since the fine print states that relapse calculations can overestimate the risk of cancer recurrence in the future and the benefit of chemotherapy or hormonal treatment.

TIP For most people, the prognosis gets better with time. Sometimes we use a five-year figure because we know that if cancer comes back, most of the time it comes back within five years. If the cancer has not come back within five years, then the chance of it coming back within ten years is quite low.

REMEMBER Doctors can only give you a guide to your prognosis; they cannot predict your future with accuracy. There are plenty of patients who have beaten the odds despite having been told they had a poor prognosis.

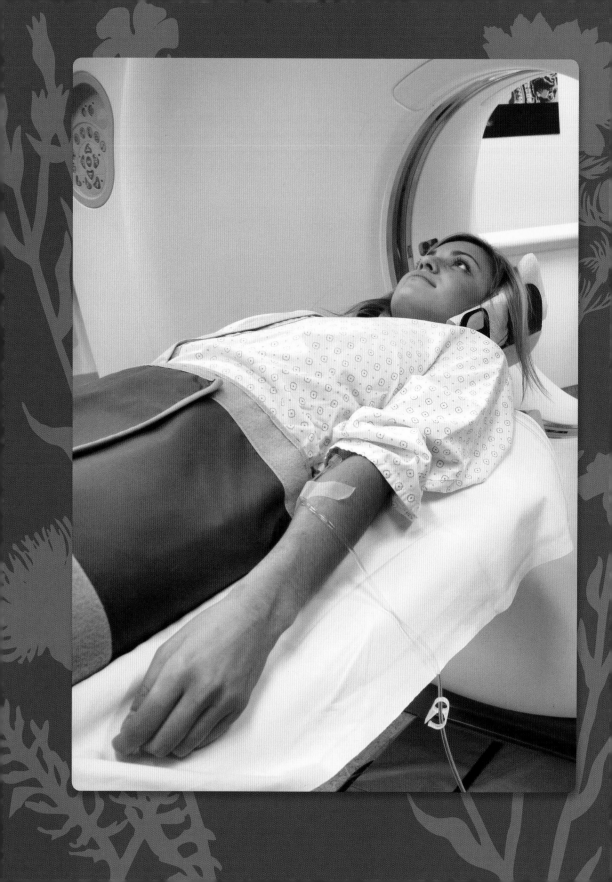

Control Point 13

Do I Need Additional Tests?

Control Point #13

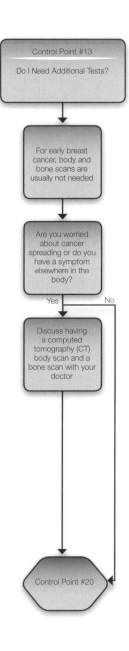

Control Point #13

Do I Need Additional Tests?

For early breast cancer, body and bone scans are usually not needed

Are you worried about cancer spreading or do you have a symptom elsewhere in the body?

Yes

No

Discuss having a computed tomography (CT) body scan and a bone scan with your doctor

Control Point #20

Do I Need Additional Tests?

Lots of tests are usually unnecessary

There is rarely a reason to do lots and lots of tests, though many doctors still order them, often unnecessarily, to see if cancer has spread to other parts of the body from the breast. For example, cancer that has spread from the breast to the bone is called "metastatic breast cancer to the bone." It is not "bone cancer" that started as a separate cancer; it's the same "weed" that has seeded another part of the garden. Scans and blood tests are helpful, however, if cancer has come back, because they may provide an easy way to check that you are responding to treatment.

The problem with tests is that you have to find large amounts of cancer to be able to see it with the types of tests that we have available today. Cancers generally have to be over 10 mm before they are seen on scans of the body.

It's better to have more tests when the chance of finding something increases. In general, we tend to perform staging tests when the cancer is more advanced, and this includes the following situations:

- When the cancer is over 50 mm in the breast

- When there are four or more lymph glands involved in the armpit

- When the tumor is "locally advanced," meaning that there are either skin changes or the cancer is attached to the muscle underneath the breast

- If you have unexplained pain or any other symptoms that may suggest that the cancer has spread.

Remember that most pains at the point of diagnosis are due to arthritis or muscular pains, and are not due to cancer. If a pain is persistent and does not go away with simple Tylenol (acetaminophen)/Panadol (paracetamol), then X-rays will be necessary. There are different ways of testing whether or not the cancer may have spread. Cancer tends to spread to organs such as the lungs or the bones or the liver, and, rarely, the brain.

In the past, we used to do some blood tests, and if the liver tests were abnormal, then we would do an ultrasound of the liver (a test using sound waves, but no radiation) and a chest X-ray. If the bone blood test was abnormal, then a **bone scan** was done. This is done on the same machine used for sentinel node mapping, but with a different dye (Figure 37).

This is still a very useful, simple approach. Today, we often find it simpler just to do a **CT scan** of the thorax (the chest), the abdomen, and the pelvis, along with a bone scan, and this picks up most abnormalities. If you have a significant headache (not just a tension headache from the stress involved following your diagnosis) or blurred vision, then we would also do a CT scan of the head.

Remember, if you have an early breast cancer, there really is no need for all these tests. They just cause more anxiety and can also result in "false positives" by picking up abnormalities that have been present all your life. I often see liver cysts visible on CT scans that are done for radiation therapy planning purposes.

Another common problem is a single spot on a bone that may be due to an old fracture or some inflammation where the rib joins the cartilage. These abnormalities are probably okay, but you can imagine the stress and often unnecessary worry they cause.

So remember, don't rush in and have tests. However, if you're going to sit there and worry about not having tests and making sure that your cancer hasn't spread, then perhaps it's easier just to get a quick chest X-ray, some blood tests, and a liver ultrasound, which doesn't expose you to too much extra radiation.

Other tests are expensive and not really necessary, too, in my opinion. Magnetic resonance imaging scans (MRI) and positron emission tomography (PET) scans of the whole body have been used in some circumstances, but they're probably best used in situations where the cancer has come back and conventional tests have been unable to identify the extent of the recurrence.

I have many patients who are told by friends to have cancer-specific blood tests. There are a whole range of these, including CEA, CA 15-3 and CA 27-29. All of these are non-specific markers found in the blood. They are really not very useful. In one clinic, for example, I saw two patients: one who was totally scared because a blood test was slightly above the normal range, though all other tests were clear; and one whose disease had come back in three different places but whose tests were perfectly normal!

The problem with most tests is that there are false negatives and false positives, and I think it is better to treat you as an individual rather than just to look at you as being well or not well by a series of tests.

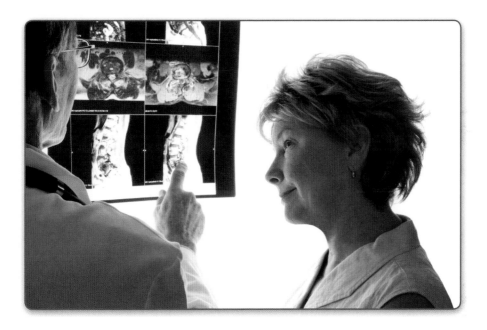

CONTROL POINT #13 – DO I NEED ADDITIONAL TESTS?

 Don't rush in and have tests. However, if you're going to sit there and worry about not having tests and making sure that your cancer hasn't spread, then perhaps it's easier to have a few quick scans.

 Cancer-specific blood tests such as CA 15-3 are not all that helpful for most patients and can be associated with false positives and false negatives.

 If your breast cancer has been picked up early, then the only tests you may need apart from your mammogram, ultrasound, and biopsies for your breast are some simple blood tests before your surgery and sometimes a chest X-ray.

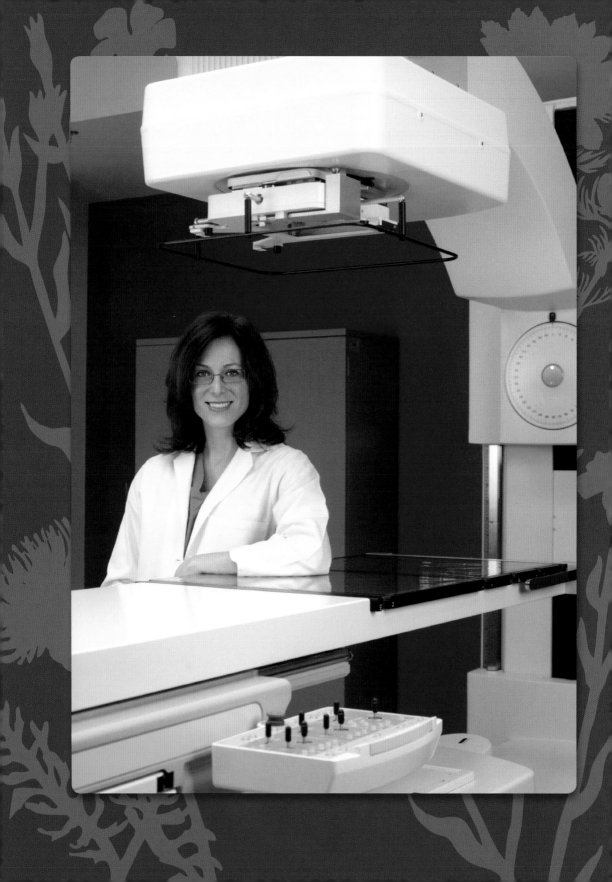

Control Point 14

Do I Need Radiation Therapy?

Control Point #14

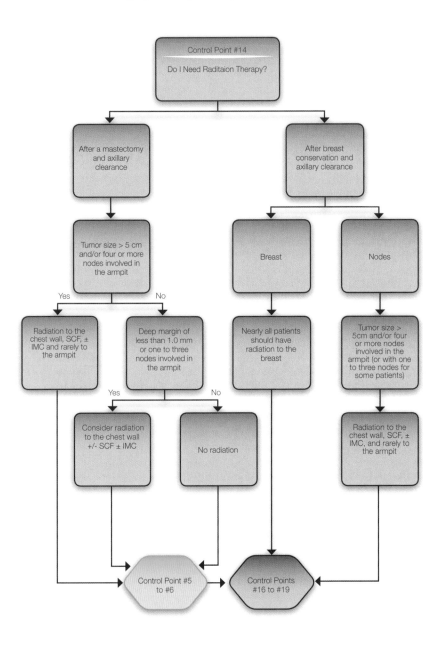

Control Point #14

Do I Need Raditaion Therapy?

After a mastectomy and axillary clearance

After breast conservation and axillary clearance

Tumor size > 5 cm and/or four or more nodes involved in the armpit

Breast

Nodes

Yes — Radiation to the chest wall, SCF, ± IMC and rarely to the armpit

No — Deep margin of less than 1.0 mm or one to three nodes involved in the armpit

Nearly all patients should have radiation to the breast

Tumor size > 5cm and/or four or more nodes involved in the armpit (or with one to three nodes for some patients)

Yes — Consider radiation to the chest wall +/- SCF ± IMC

No — No radiation

Radiation to the chest wall, SCF, ± IMC, and rarely to the armpit

Control Point #5 to #6

Control Points #16 to #19

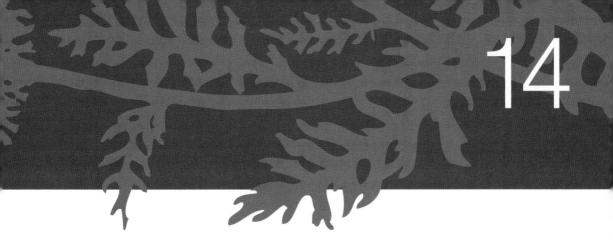

Do I Need Radiation Therapy?

What is radiation therapy?

There is no doubt that you may not really "hear" what the doctor is saying if you're suddenly hit with words like, "You now need chemotherapy/radiation therapy." You may not even have been warned about this possibility before your surgery.

Radiation therapy basically uses radiation to destroy cancer cells. There are many different forms of radiation, but the most common type used to treat women with breast cancer is what we call **external-beam radiation**. Radiation is produced when electrons are shot between a cathode (usually made of copper) and an anode (usually made of tungsten).

In the late afternoon of November 8, 1895, Wilhelm Röntgen discovered this magical beam, a ray that was unknown, or "x." Although these special rays were named after him, he always preferred to call them X-rays. Very soon after the discovery of radiation, it was found that it was able to destroy cancer cells because they're more sensitive to radiation than normal cells, such as your skin cells.

Radiation therapy damages the DNA or genetic material of cells in the area being treated, stopping these cells from growing and dividing. Although radiation damages both cancer cells and normal cells, most normal cells can recover within a few hours because they have all the repair mechanisms present to do so, whereas cancer cells, because they are abnormal, can't repair themselves as well. Radiation given after surgery is called "adjuvant" radiation.

Radiation therapy to the whole breast after breast conservation

A very common question I'm asked is, "Why do I need to have radiation to my breast after a lumpectomy when I'm having chemotherapy anyway?" This is a very good, logical question. For some reason, chemotherapy or hormonal treatment alone is not enough. I sometimes wonder whether it's because surgery has disrupted the blood supply to the area, thus making it harder for the chemotherapy the get to the point where the cancer started (the "**tumor bed**"). My other theory is that because what's left behind is mostly pre-cancer or DCIS, chemotherapy really doesn't work because the cells it's treating aren't cancer yet. Radiation therapy, on the other hand, has been shown to work for both invasive cancer and pre-cancerous DCIS.

If we look at my garden example again, giving radiotherapy to your breast after a lumpectomy, is like putting a weed mat or straw mulch down after you remove a weed from under a rose bush (Figure 25). Even though the soil looks clear, some seeds may have been left behind, and the weed can come back again.

I won't go into too much detail on partial breast irradiation, except to say that it's best to do this if you're in a clinical trial situation and will be closely monitored. Theoretically, at least, not treating the whole breast will increase the risk of breast cancer coming back in other parts of the breast, but this could be a reasonable option if you're older, have a low-grade cancer that is easily seen on a mammogram, and have difficulty accessing five to six weeks of radiation. The American College of Breast Surgeons recommends limiting this treatment to a trial setting, and outside of a trial recommends restricting this practice to patients who:

- Are age 45 or older
- Have invasive ductal carcinoma or DCIS
- Have a total tumor size (invasive and DCIS) of less than or equal to 30 mm
- Have clear margins under the microscope
- Have no involved axillary lymph glands.

Table 9 shows the 20-year results from the most important breast conservation trial to date, performed by US physician Bernard Fisher (Fisher 2002). Remember that these results were from over 30 years ago, when mammography and breast ultrasound were virtually non-existent or very rudimentary, so the true extent of disease was often underestimated.

Nearly half of all patients (44%) in the group with node positive breast cancer treated with a lumpectomy followed by chemotherapy had their cancer come back in their breast. Patients whose lymph glands were not involved ("node negative") who had a lumpectomy without radiation therapy also had a high risk of the cancer coming back in the breast (36%) which was still nearly four in ten. When radiation was added, the risk of the breast cancer coming back was about 1 percent every year (17 percent at 20 years).

	Node-Negative (no chemotherapy)	Node-Positive (chemotherapy)
Lumpectomy Only	36%	44%
Lumpectomy and Radiation	17%	9%

Table 9: Chance of cancer coming back in the breast after breast conservation with a lumpectomy

When chemotherapy was combined with radiation therapy for women with node-positive breast cancer, the results were even better with only a 9% chance of recurrence in the breast, suggesting that the two help each other or are "synergistic." We have found this holds true for many different types of cancers.

Some of my own research has shown that the risk of breast cancer coming back in the breast after a lumpectomy and radiation therapy decreased as you got older (Leong 2004). Very young women (aged 34 years or younger at diagnosis) had a slightly higher chance of the cancer coming back, even when the margins were clear, and older women had a lower risk, even when the margins were close or positive.

Ultimately, what we're trying to do is to ensure that there's only a small or no tumor burden left behind that we can get rid of by radiation therapy.

Radiation therapy after a mastectomy

It can be frustrating when you've gone through the trauma of having your breast removed, and for all intents and purposes the cancer is "gone", and your wound has healed, and the doctor says, "You need to have radiation therapy." This can be very distressing and feels at first like a major setback.

Radiation therapy to the chest wall has been used since the late '60s and early '70s. In the early trials from the UK, patients were treated with what was called a **simple mastectomy**. It was called "simple" because in those days, a "radical mastectomy" involved removing the breast, the pectoralis major and minor muscles, and the skin of the chest wall, and this usually involved a skin graft from the thigh. The simple mastectomy removed the breast without all the muscles or the lymph glands under the armpit.

This radical mastectomy was first preached by a surgeon from New York, William S. Halsted, who was named the first chief of the Department of Surgery at Johns Hopkins Hospital when it opened in May 1889. Halsted would not be too impressed today that we have replaced his "radical" disfiguring procedure with a lumpectomy and radiation therapy. It was quite a horrendous operation, which left women with significant psychological and physical side effects.

A famous Scottish radiation oncologist called McWhirter introduced a trial of a simple mastectomy and radiation therapy and compared this to a radical mastectomy. Very soon, it became clear that the extent of surgery didn't really change someone's prognosis when radiation therapy was added.

Even though there was nothing "simple" about this mastectomy, (the poor woman still lost all her breast), it was a first attempt to try to reduce the amount of surgery, and was the beginning of an understanding that although local treatments are very important, the extent of the surgery and radiation therapy could be modified to improve a woman's quality of life.

The next generation of studies then looked at what was called a "**total mastectomy** and axillary dissection," and compared this to the same treatment with or without radiation therapy. The regional lymph glands included the lymph glands above the breastbone (the supra-clavicular or "SCF" nodes), sometimes the glands in the armpit (axilla), and sometimes the lymph glands found just beside the breastbone (the internal mammary chain or "IMC") (Figure 35).

These studies (where treatment was decided almost by a toss of the coin; "heads," women had a mastectomy alone and "tails," they had mastectomy and radiation therapy) showed that for many patients, there was actually a survival advantage to reducing the chance of cancer coming back over the chest wall or in the region of the glands.

For many years, it was thought that reducing the chance of cancer coming back "locally" (in the breast, chest wall, or lymph glands) didn't really matter. But the latest studies have found that optimizing local control does improve survival rates by at least 5 to 10 percent.

You would think that it was common sense to reduce the chance of cancer coming back, but in the '70s and '80s, there were a lot of women who just received a mastectomy and chemotherapy, and often patients were not given the much-needed additional local therapy such as radiation therapy to the chest wall or the breast.

Chances of recurrence after a mastectomy and axillary dissection, with and without radiation therapy

In 1997, I published a paper called "Post-Mastectomy Radiation Therapy: Better Late than Never," in which we summarized the just-published trials from Denmark and Canada that proved that radiation therapy after a mastectomy improved survival.

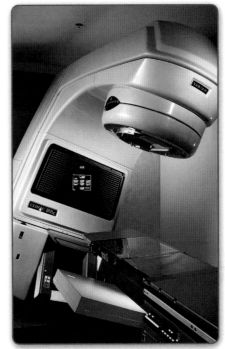

Figure 73: A modern linear accelerator, which delivers radiotherapy treatment.

At the same time, we looked at the long-term recurrence rates on the chest wall or lymph gland areas in patients who were treated with a total mastectomy, axillary dissection, and chemotherapy without radiation therapy. The results are summarized below (Table 10) (Langlands 1997). The trials had an average follow-up time of about ten and 12 years for the Danish and Canadian trials, and eight years for our study.

So basically, at least for patients treated in the '80s with a total mastectomy and what we now call "first generation" chemotherapy (which I will explain later), the recurrence rates on the chest wall or lymph glands were fairly low if a woman had a

Number of Involved Lymph Glands	Pathologic Tumor Size		
	Up to 20 mm	21–50 mm	> 50 mm
1–3 Nodes	7%	13%	46%
4–10 Nodes	38%	23%	75%

Table 10: Study showing the chance of cancer coming back in the chest wall or lymph glands after a mastectomy

tumor that measured up to 20 mm or 21–50mm with one to three glands involved in the armpit (7% and 13% respectively). But if a woman had a T3 tumor (measured 50 mm or more on her microscopic pathology report) or if she had four or more nodes involved, the recurrence rates were quite substantial ranging from 23% to 75%. Although the rates for a local recurrence were higher for patients with tumors up to 20 mm and 4–10 nodes (38%) than for those with tumors 21–50 mm (23%), this was probably due to the fact that there were very few patients with tumors up to 20 mm, and thus the statistics were less accurate in this group.

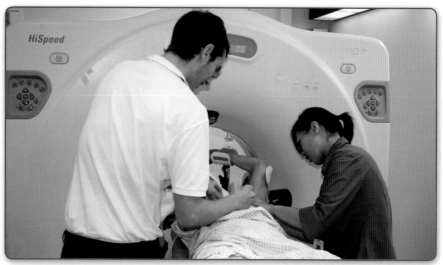
Figure 74: A CT scan is done during the radiation therapy planning procedure.

The results from the Canadian and Denmark trials showed that in patients with four or more lymph glands involved, the average recurrence rate in the chest wall or surrounding nodal areas was about 30 percent without radiation therapy and 15 percent with radiation therapy. A very large **meta-analysis** looked at the results of 8,500 women who had a mastectomy with or without subsequent radiation. Fifteen years after treatment, the investigators reported that women with cancer in their lymph glands had an average loco-regional recurrence rate of 23 percent without radiation, compared to 6 percent with radiation, and an improvement in survival rates of 5 percent.

In other words, radiation can reduce the risk of breast cancer coming back in the chest wall or the surrounding glands by about 75%. This is not trivial and it's therefore worth talking to your surgeon about the chance of your cancer coming back with or without radiation. The good news is that modern hormonal treatments can also reduce the risk of cancer coming back in the chest wall and glands, but probably not as permanently as radiation. The authors reported that for every four recurrences in the chest wall or gland areas prevented, one life was saved (Early Breast Cancer Trialists' Collaborative Group 2005).

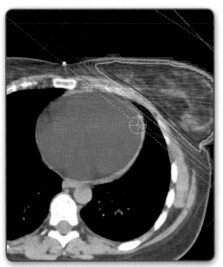
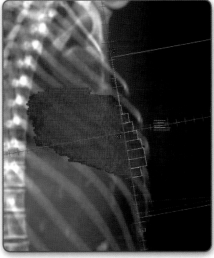

Figure 75: A radiation therapy plan is calculated specifically for your body using powerful 3D computers.

When is radiation therapy given?

If no other treatments, such as chemotherapy, are to be given, then radiation therapy usually starts three to six weeks after surgery. This is provided that you can lift your arm above your head to get it out of the way and allow the radiation to target your breast or chest wall, and that all surgical wounds have healed. Normally, hormonal drugs are given after the radiation is completed (Figure 86, treatment strategy A and I). If chemotherapy is given, radiation normally starts about three weeks after your last course (Figure 86, treatment strategies B to G, L to P and R).

Where is radiation therapy given?

In general, radiation therapy is given to the breast or chest wall and the lymph glands at the base of the neck (SCF glands). We sometimes treat the armpit if there is extensive disease present, such as if cancer extends from the gland into the surrounding fat (extranodal spread). We sometimes treat the lymph glands behind the breastbone, but this varies between treatment centers. Most centers agree to give radiation to the breast after a lumpectomy, and to the chest wall when the tumor in the breast measured larger than 50 mm on the pathology report, or when four or more lymph glands were involved in the armpit. There is increasing evidence that treating patients with one to three lymph glands involved in the armpit is beneficial, but this is still being investigated in clinical trials. I consider radiation when there is extensive lymphatic invasion around the cancer, when there are multiple tumors which add up to over 40 to 50 mm, when the margin between the cancer and the chest wall is less than one millimeter, or if there is cancer in the gland behind the breastbone (the internal mammary chain (IMC) lymph gland).

How is radiation therapy given?

A standard **linear accelerator** is used to produce and accurately deliver the radiation to your breast area (Figure 73). It looks scary, but don't be afraid of it. It doesn't hurt, and all you need to do is lie still and breathe in and out normally. It's a fairly open machine in a large room, and not too claustrophobic. The machine is used by specially trained staff called **radiation therapists** or radiation technologists who position you carefully every day. Your position is based on the prescription and plan approved by your radiation oncologist. While the radiation beam is turned on, they can see and hear you through a closed-circuit television. The actual time it takes to give the radiation to each area is usually less than a minute, but each treatment slot may be ten to 15 minutes long because of the time it takes to position you accurately using coordinates determined at the planning process.

How much radiation is given?

Radiation therapy is given daily (five days per week or sometimes five days one week and four days the next) for about five to six weeks. The standard dose of radiation given each day is 1.8 to 2.0 units. The amount of radiation absorbed by the tissues is called the radiation dose (called a **gray**, or Gy). Some doctors still use the imperial measure, called a rad. One Gy is equal to 100 **rads**. After breast conservation, various dose prescriptions are given by different doctors. A common dose used for the whole breast in the US and Australia is 50 Gy over the course of 25 sessions (also called "**fractions**"). Shorter courses of radiation, over three weeks, are commonly used in Canada and the UK (Whelan 2010) After the first 50 Gy, there is usually an extra week of radiation, at a dose of 2 Gy per day for five days. This is called a **boost**, and it's given to the tumor bed because this is where most recurrences in the breast tend to occur. A large clinical trial in Europe proved that women who received a boost had a lower recurrence rate than those who did not (Poortmans 2008). Remember:

- You are not radioactive and you can continue to hug and kiss your partner and your children
- You will not glow in the dark nor "beep" when you go through airport security!
- You are not more susceptible to infections
- You can continue to work
- You need to attend somewhere between 16 and 33 treatments
- You will not "beep" when you You can drive to and from treatment.

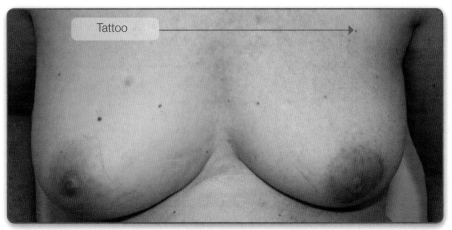

Figure 76: Skin reddening after week four of radiation to the left breast. A tattoo is used to guide treatment.

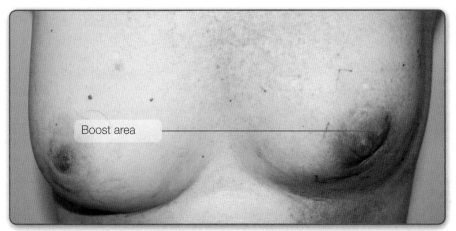

Figure 77: Skin reddening, six weeks after radiation, becoming worse over the scar ("boost").

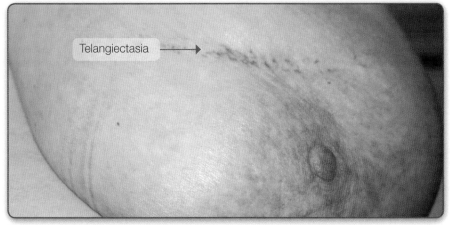

Figure 78: Prominent red marks, called "telangiectasia," over the scar ten years after treatment.

The radiation therapy planning session

This first visit can be quite scary. Obviously, the doctors and the technicians go through this every day, and hopefully they are sensitive to your fears (Figure 74). I usually let a patient's partner go in to the room to be with them for part of the planning procedure. At this planning session, which is also called a **simulation**, I always like to look at mammograms to see how big the breast cancer was so that we can work out where to give the extra "boost" dose of radiation. Make sure you bring your X-rays along with you.

Most radiation therapy departments mark your skin with some permanent marks (tattoos) using a small amount of ink and a pinprick (Figure 76). The number of tattoos varies between departments but usually range between three and six. Some departments avoid using a the tattoo in the area of the neckline, which does make wearing low tops after radiation a little easier. Tattoos do fade with time and can be covered easily with cosmetic creams after treatment, or in rare circumstances, one that may be particularly bothersome to you can be surgically removed.

Many modern departments have what is called a CT simulator, and a CT scan is done right then and there. (A CT is sometimes referred to as a "CAT scan" (Figure 74). The visit to the simulator will take about 30 minutes. A planning CT scan is exactly the same as a diagnostic CT scan. You lie on a bed, and it takes X-ray "slices" of your body from around the middle of your neck to about 2–3 cm under your breast.

These slices are used to recreate a three-dimensional image of your upper body using a modern supercomputer. The radiation doctor (radiotherapist or radiation oncologist) can mark where the cancer started, where your breast is, and where vital organs such as the lung, heart, and spinal cord are located. Most of the planning work takes place behind the scenes over the next week using very complex mathematics done by a radiation therapist who specializes in computerized planning (such therapists are called **dosimetrists** or radiation therapy planners in some countries); this is why you may have to wait so long between your planning appointment and your first treatment. Figure 75 shows a typical radiation plan showing shielding of the heart.

Today we can restrict the amount of involved lung under your breast to small amounts. A small amount of involved lung is required to ensure that we don't under-treat the part of your breast that sits on your ribs just above your lung. I think it is also important to minimize the amount of radiation that your heart gets. Sometimes it's simply not possible, but most times with modern three-dimensional radiation therapy, it's possible to protect all of the heart with special shields called multileaf collimators.

It's not always easy, though, so don't be too hard on your radiation oncologist. Some women have barrel chests and have more lung in the field than normal. Other women's hearts might be big because of early heart failure. Sometimes the location of the cancer makes it impossible to totally miss the heart, particularly when it's in the lower outer part of your left breast (i.e., the 4 to 5 o'clock position) or when it is located right next to the breastbone on the left side. It is really important to make sure that the cancer is treated properly, and if it means some unavoidable radiation to the heart, don't get too worried—the risk of heart damage is still very low.

Particularly if you're under age 55 and are having lots of chemotherapy or Herceptin, which can also upset the heart, just ask, "What dose is my heart receiving?" or "How much heart is in the field? Can I have a look at the where the path of the X-ray beam is going and where my heart is?" or, "Can the lower part of my heart be shielded?"

Common side effects during radiation therapy

Tiredness

You may feel tired during the treatment, particularly in the later weeks. Nobody really knows if it's just the radiation that causes this; a lot of my patients don't sleep all that well during this treatment because of the stress of the diagnosis and getting used to the fact that life has changed for the moment. Exercise may help with your tiredness, and sometimes a multivitamin, although this is controversial.

Aches and pains in the breast

You may feel minor twinges in the breast for some time, often years. These are frequently sharp pains, usually in the scar. In my view, this is probably due to the nerves under the skin rejoining and causing some small electric shocks. There's not much you can do about this, apart from rubbing some vitamin E cream into your scar. Rest assured, though, that this will usually improve with time.

Swelling of the breast

You may develop some fluid in the breast after your surgery and radiation treatment. This is called breast edema. Edema of the breast is particularly noticeable if you wear an underwire bra, where you may see an indentation of your skin. This is not dangerous. The areola area can become thickened with the edema too, and may feel more leathery and become paler. Again, nothing to worry about. Breast lymphedema is not dangerous unless your breast gets infected and appears red and hot. If this occurs, see your doctor for some antibiotics.

Breast edema is particularly common for women with large breasts, and is worse in the first year after treatment, but it slowly improves by the third year. As with lymphedema of the arm, it is helpful to keep the breast moisturized. Some lymphedema therapists can train you to massage the fluid in the breast toward the breastbone, and this sometimes reduces the swelling.

Skin reddening and irritation

There may be some skin reddening by the second, but more usually the third or fourth, week of treatment (Figure 76), which will become brisker by week six (Figure 77). The reddening may become a little worse over the area given the boost or extra dose in the week after the treatment finishes. This often occurs toward the breastbone and sometimes your outer nipple area, as these areas receive a slightly higher dose of radiation therapy. I recommend rubbing some bland barrier cream, such as vitamin E or even aloe vera, onto the skin on a daily basis.

After your course of therapy, it's not unusual for your breast skin to become slightly darker (particularly for people with darker skin). In the longer term, a few prominent blood vessels may appear in areas of skin that received a higher dose of radiation, and this is called **telangiectasia** (Figure 78). It is not dangerous.

Loss of hair

You will not lose the hair on your head, but if your armpit region receives radiation therapy, you may lose the hair in that location, possibly permanently.

Sore throat

Sometimes when we treat the lymph glands above the breastbone, you may get a sore throat toward the end of or just after treatment. If this occurs, eat soft, non-spicy, and warm (rather than hot) foods until this settles down. Tylenol (acetaminophen) / Panadol (paracetamol) syrup may help.

Uncommon side effects during radiation therapy

Skin reactions

Toward the end of the treatment, you may experience some blisters on your skin. These usually occur only in areas that have received a slightly higher dose. When you look at the radiation therapy plan, it's like a weather map with high and low dose areas. Apart from the nipple area, other areas that can get irritated more than others are those where skin folds rub against each other, such as under your breast or in the armpit.

Modern radiation normally spares the skin, and the highest dose is about 15 mm under the skin. In some situations when we need to enhance the dose to the skin with tissue equivalent material (called bolus), the maximum dose is on the skin. This is done deliberately if we are worried about the cancer coming back on the chest wall after a mastectomy. The skin can get quite red in this situation, like bad sunburn, but it always settles down in two to four weeks.

Nausea

Nausea is quite uncommon. Radiation nausea tends to occur two to four hours after your treatment. You may feel queasy but rarely sick with radiation delivered just to the breast or chest area. If you are receiving radiation therapy to multiple areas, or if you're unlucky enough to have breast cancer in both your breasts, then this extra dose of radiation can cause radiation nausea.

If radiation nausea occurs, see your doctor about taking an anti-emetic (anti-nausea) pill half an hour before your radiation treatment. Nausea and vomiting is more of a problem with chemotherapy than with radiation therapy. Drugs used to prevent nausea and vomiting include prochlorperazine (Stemetil) or metoclopramide (Maxeran, Nabilone, Maxolon).

If you are receiving radiation therapy to other parts of your body and experience more severe nausea, then there are new agents such as ondansetron (Zofran) to help control it.

Rib problems

Rib fractures are very rare, but very occasionally a woman may get a fracture in the treated area. More often than not, it's just tenderness over the ribs. I find that a lot of women develop what is known as costochondritis, common symptoms of which include sudden, severe pain and soreness, usually around the breastbone. Pain of costochondritis increases when pressure is applied to the tender area where the cartilage connects the ribs, and also increases with coughing, sneezing, or deep breathing, all of which move the cartilage or the ribs (Figure 35).

If a rib fracture does occur, this can be diagnosed by a bone scan or an X-ray or both, and it usually happens 12 to 48 months after radiation therapy. On a nuclear bone scan, the ribs may show up as an abnormal "hot spot" indicating increased bone activity, often in a straight line in the region between the edge of your breast and your armpit. The important thing to remember is that it's very rare to get bone cancer that's spread from the breast in an area that's already had radiation therapy.

Note: some doctors may believe that this is cancer, as they may not know that you've had radiation therapy to the area. If in doubt, a CT scan with "bone windows" or "bone settings" may clarify the situation.

Rib fractures nearly always heal and are not a serious complication. Both costochondritis and rib fractures can be helped with rest, warm compresses, and the use of anti-inflammatory medications (such as aspirin, ibuprofen, naproxen, or ketoprofen).

Lung inflammation

In order to treat the breast, a small amount of lung needs to be treated so that we don't under-dose the back of your breast. The whole breast needs to be treated, either by removing it or by giving all of it radiation therapy. Lung inflammation, known as "radiation pneumonitis", is rare after treatment. One or two women in every 100 may develop lung inflammation, usually six weeks to six months after therapy. It is more common if you have had chemotherapy as well as radiation therapy. Symptoms include coughing and shortness of breath. A telltale sign is that you may feel excessively tired.

Long-term scarring can occur, but only in a very small area of the lung. More lung is exposed when we need to treat the lymph glands above the breastbone or the supraclavicular fossa.

All doctors treat this a little differently and one size doesn't fit all. This is what I do:

- Perform a chest X-ray (and sometimes a CT scan) to confirm that nothing else is going on

- Start some antibiotics, usually just simple Augmentin (amoxicillin, 500 mg, four times a day)

- Commence prednisone at a dose of 20 mg a day and reduce the dose by half every three days.

Other cancers

Women who have had radiation therapy may be susceptible to other cancers. There is a slightly increased risk of ovarian cancer, for example, if there is a family history of breast cancer, which may indicate genetic susceptibility to breast and ovarian cancer. This is not due to the radiation therapy.

Sometimes, body fat breaks down around the scar, and when the fat dies and liquefies, this is called "fat necrosis." The body can calcify this area, and sometimes it may look like a recurrence, but it is nothing to worry about.

Very rarely, radiation may cause cancer. This is known as a **sarcoma** and can even occur after a mastectomy. Estimates vary, but one study reported nine cases of sarcoma in 20,000 women treated over a 20 year period usually five to nine years after treatment (Marchal 1999). But remember, this is like winning the lottery. I have seen three cases in 25 years. Assume it won't be you.

It's important to do a biopsy of any new tumors in the breast, particularly when they occur in the second five years, to exclude this more serious type of cancer. A recent report suggested a slightly higher risk of lung cancer if you have radiation for breast cancer (Candace and Darby 2009). More research is needed, but if you smoke, try to stop or at least cut back.

Excessive shrinkage of the breast

About one in 1000 women may be more sensitive to radiation, and the breast may shrink quite substantially. There is really no way to know if this will happen. It tends to be more of a problem for women with larger-breasts. If this occurs, plastic surgery may be able to help. Very rarely, a mastectomy will need to be done. The more common situation is shown in Figure 79. This is a photograph seven years after radiation showing how the other breast sags with time particularly if you put on weight. There is a slight amount of persistent pigmentation over the scar, and

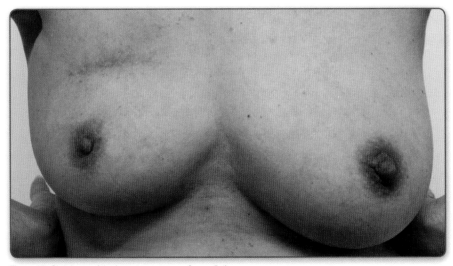

Figure 79: Shrinkage of the breast can occur after radiation.

shrinkage of the treated right breast made worse by gaining weight and depositing fat in the untreated breast but not the treated breast.

Pain in the breast

Often, there are sharp or shooting pains, usually over the scar. They don't last long, but may give you a bit of a scare. Sometimes a supporting bra helps these. Rubbing vitamin E cream into the scar may help in the longer term. These pains may occur in as many as seven out of ten women.

Nerve damage

Treatment to the lymph glands above the breastbone or clavicle can in very rare circumstances produce damage to the nerves that start at the neck and go to the arm and hand. Damage to this nerve bundle, called the brachial plexus, can occur a few years after radiation and may be temporary or permanent. This can cause numbness and tingling or even loss of power in some or all of the hand. It is important that this area is treated slowly over five weeks using no more than two units of radiation a day. With modern radiation therapy planning, this is very, very rare, and most oncologists may only see one or two cases in their career.

Breast feeding

After breast conservation, breast feeding is usually not possible on the side where radiation was given, although a small amount of fluid may discharge from the nipple. Usually, the treated side stays smaller and the untreated side becomes larger and droops more as your pregnancy progresses. There is no problem with breast feeding from your untreated breast, provided you are not having chemotherapy.

Tenderness over the pectoral muscle

Sometimes women get pain over the pectoralis (pec) muscles. The pec can be found by holding the muscle at the front of your armpit. These pains are not uncommon and are usually caused by some scarring of the muscle from radiation therapy. Because the pectoralis muscle is close to the surface, it does receive a slightly higher dose of radiation, and this can sometimes cause some discomfort and lack of mobility. Massage of the area by a physical therapist may help, as may rubbing vitamin E cream into the area regularly and continuing your shoulder exercises.

Skin care during and after your radiation therapy

This will vary according to your local treatment team. What you can do for yourself includes the following:

- Use a very mild soap, such as baby soap

- Use warm water when you shower or bathe instead of very hot water

- After showering, pat the skin dry rather than rub

- Simple barrier creams such as Sorbolene (Australia, UK), vitamin E cream, or Eucerin are helpful. Do not use creams that contain excessive cosmetics or perfumes. Rub the Sorbolene cream into your treated area every day after treatment.

At the beginning of treatment, before you have any side effects, moisturize the skin after your daily treatment with an ointment such as A&D, Eucerin, Aquaphor, Biafene, Sorbolene, vitamin E or Radiacare. You also can put it on at night—wear an old t-shirt so the ointment doesn't get on your bedclothes. I recommend you do this only after your daily treatment, as sometimes the radiation therapy technicians need to add a few more marks to your skin just before treatment, and this may be difficult if your skin is slippery with cream.

Here are a few more tips:

- For mild pinkness, itching, and burning, apply an aloe vera preparation. Or try 0.5% to 1% hydrocortisone cream (usually available without a prescription at any drugstore). Spread the cream thinly over the affected area three times a day.

- If areas become red, itchy, sore, and start to burn, and low-potency cream no longer relieves your symptoms, ask your doctor for a stronger steroid cream available by prescription. Examples include 2.5% hydrocortisone cream and betamethasone.

- Some women get some relief by blowing air on the area with a hair dryer set to "cool" or "air." Don't turn it to "heat."

- Don't wear a bra if there are raw areas, unless you cover them with some burn cream and a pad. If your skin forms a blister or peels in a wet way, leave the top of the blister alone! The bubble keeps the area clean while the new skin grows back underneath. If the blister opens, the exposed raw area can be painful and weepy. Keep the area relatively dry and wash it with warm water only. Blot the area dry and then apply a non-adherent dressing, such as Xeroform or "second skin" dressings. To relieve any discomfort you can take an over-the-counter pain reliever.

- I normally do not recommend aluminum-based deodorants during radiation therapy. There are some natural deodorants around, including tea tree oil and a product called rock salt. Again, this is probably just a myth, but theoretically, the aluminum in the deodorants may interact with the radiation therapy and cause a more severe skin reaction. Talk to your local pharmacist about what's available in your country. However, if it's the middle of summer and the natural deodorants are not working, perhaps a spray deodorant may be the best approach.

- Do not shave under the arm with a razor blade on the treated side. You can use an electric shaver. The problem with shaving is that it can introduce infection with very superficial skin cuts.

- If radiation therapy is given to the armpit area, the sweat glands can become dry and some patients stop sweating on that side. Sometimes the hair doesn't grow back. Many women think this is a bonus! Apply a barrier cream to the areas of dry skin.

- Speak to your breast care nurse about the best bra to use. There are bra specialists that can help you. Cotton bras are probably better than nylon bras, as the nylon can irritate the nipple area (Figure 52). Sometimes just putting a large cotton handkerchief between the bra and your breasts will help. Many find wearing a bra towards the end of treatment is too abrasive and causes too much rubbing over sensitive skin.

- Cotton t-shirts or singlets are helpful. Some women prefer not to wear a bra, particularly if they have small breasts. If you have large-breasts, good support is necessary, and sometimes a sports bra is helpful.

- For women wih large-breasts, sometimes the fold between your breast and your abdomen rubs just from the normal bounce of the breast, and this can be an area of irritation from friction. Putting a pad (such as sanitary pad or a Telfa® pad) between your bra and your skin may help to protect this area, as may applying some paw paw gel (derived from the papaya tree, if available in your country), aloe vera, or creams such as Eucerin, Lubriderm, or Aquaphor. If you're having treatment in the area above the breastbone, the radiation can "exit" through your upper back and that area can become itchy. Make sure you rub Sorbolene cream into the area above your breastbone and also around the top of your back.

- If the skin peels, there are special creams used by the radiation therapy department. They do vary, but they include superficial burn creams (SSD cream, Solugel, or paw paw). Some of these creams need a dressing on top as they are quite sticky, but they are soothing.

- Don't expose your treated skin to extreme temperatures. Avoid hot water bottles, electric blankets or ice packs.

- A short swim in salt water is usually no problem during radiation therapy but chlorinated water may irritate the skin. If you do take a swim in your pool, keep it short and pad yourself dry with a soft towel.

- After treatment, continue to moisturize the skin of your breast, chest wall, and arm at least once a day if possible.

- You will need to use sun protection cream or wear a sun protection t-shirt. Minimize sun exposure in the middle of the day and make sure you wear protective clothing, sunglasses and a broad-brimmed hat.

- However, it's important not to wrap yourself up in cotton wool; try to get back to normal as quickly as possible.

As mentioned, much of this advice does vary from center to center, and it's important to talk to your own treatment team about their specific recommendations. Although it may be daunting at first, radiation treatment is usually over fairly quickly. One of my patients once explained that radiation is like a six-week vacation: before you know it, it's over and you're back at work.

CONTROL POINT #14 – DO I NEED RADIATION THERAPY?

 WARNING Treatment of your cancer with a lumpectomy *without* radiation increases your chances of the cancer coming back in the breast and may reduce your chance of cure. Always make sure you seek the opinion of a radiation oncologist as well as a surgeon.

 TIP You may feel minor twinges in the breast for some time, often for years, particularly around your scar. They are not a sign that the cancer has come back.

 REMEMBER Radiation therapy after breast conservation has been proven to be just as effective as a mastectomy, provided that clear margins are achieved after your surgery.

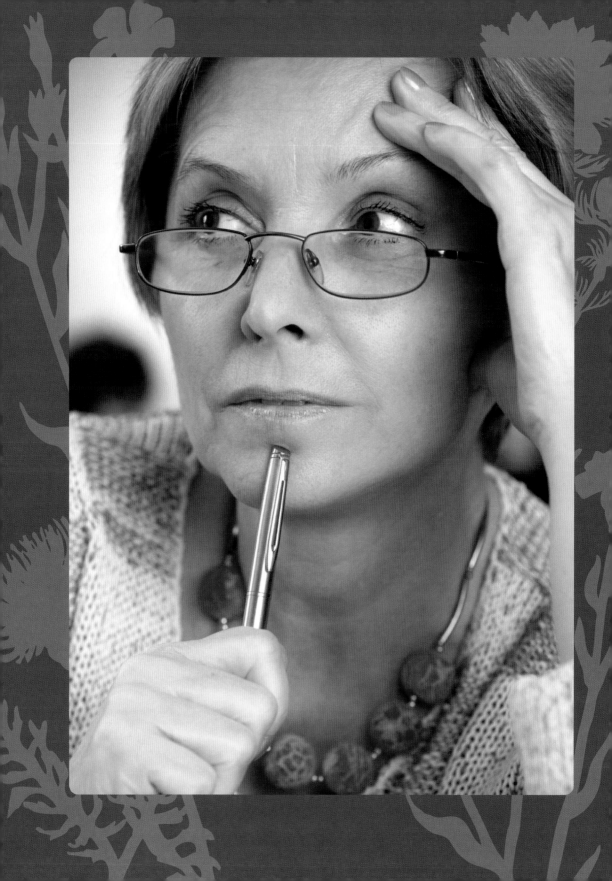

Control Point 15

What Do the Statistics Really Mean?

Control Point #15

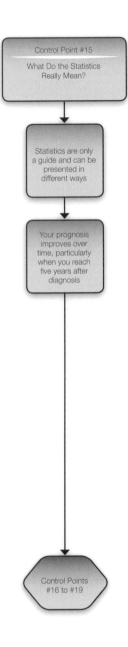

Control Point #15

What Do the Statistics Really Mean?

Statistics are only a guide and can be presented in different ways

Your prognosis improves over time, particularly when you reach five years after diagnosis

Control Points #16 to #19

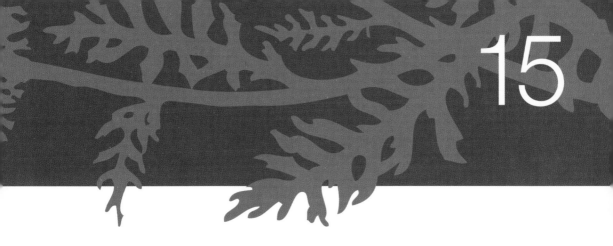

What Do the Statistics Really Mean?

Another garden analogy

Once your pathology report is available, one of the difficult decisions you may have to face is the prospect of chemotherapy and, to a lesser extent, hormonal treatment. Understanding how doctors use statistics will help you take control of the often very difficult decision about chemotherapy.

Let's go back to my gardening example for a moment. When we look at a particular weed under the rose bush (the breast), we can sometimes predict whether it's a type of weed that can blow in the wind and land in another part of the garden. If it's a fragile onion weed or dandelion, then it's more likely to seed than a broad leaf weed that tends to stay in the one place. The same applies for the different breast cancers that we can see under a microscope.

A grade 3 tumor, for example, is more fragile and more likely to blow in the wind than a grade 1 tumor. This doesn't happen in all people, but when it does, research has shown that giving treatments that treat the whole body can result in better cure rates than just having treatment to your breast.

Chemotherapy or hormonal treatment are like giving weed killer to the rest of the garden, just in case a seed has blown to another part of the body (Figure 80). Sometimes this weed killer does not discriminate very well between the weed and the good plants and damage can occur. Similarly, chemotherapy not only kills the bad cells but can damage the good cells as well.

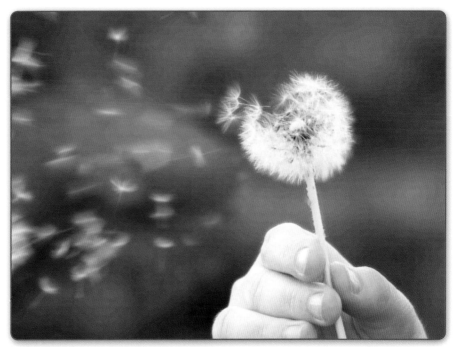

Figure 80: An important question is whether we need to use "weed killer" for another part of the garden, particularly if your cancer is grade 3 and more likely to spread "seeds" elsewhere in the body.

In this book, I will not talk about all the reasons we use chemotherapy. We sometimes use it as the initial, pre-surgical treatment (neo-adjuvant) for larger breast cancers to shrink them down and make surgery easier, particularly if a woman really wants to keep her breast. We also use it for larger cancers, which we call "locally advanced cancer"; and we certainly use it for some patients whose cancer has spread to other parts of the body.

Understanding the statistical language

Table 11 shows two hypothetical situations. Angela and Mary are both aged 50. Angela has a cancer with a lot of lymph glands involved. Let's assume her ten-year survival rate without chemotherapy is 60 percent. This means that her mortality rate (the chance of dying) from breast cancer is 40 percent. Now let's assume that she has chemotherapy with a one-quarter (25 percent) "risk reduction" in her mortality rate. One quarter of the mortality rate of 40 percent is 10 percent.

Mary, on the other hand, has a 92 percent ten-year survival rate without chemotherapy and an 8 percent mortality rate from her breast cancer. Let's assume that giving chemotherapy reduces the risk of dying by the same 25 percent. This 25 percent figure is known as a "proportional reduction," or "risk reduction," or "an odds ratio."

Patient	10-year survival without chemotherapy	Risk reduction with chemotherapy	Absolute benefit of chemotherapy	10-year survival with chemotherapy
Angela	60%	25%	10%	70%
Mary	92%	25%	2%	94%

Table 11: Understanding what all the percentages mean

It does not mean that your chances are reduced by 25 percent if you don't have chemotherapy. With chemotherapy, a 25 percent reduction means a one-quarter reduction in the death rate. The death rate for Mary was 8 percent, and a one-quarter reduction is 2 percent.

This is a very important concept to understand. Some oncologists quote the proportional reduction and almost talk you into having chemotherapy. Why wouldn't you take a 25 percent improvement? However, Mary has a 92 percent chance of cure without chemotherapy and a 94 percent with chemotherapy. If her tumor is hormone sensitive, her benefit with just hormonal treatment may be close to 2 percent without the need to lose her hair and the more difficult side effects of chemotherapy, including nausea, vomiting, and effects on the skin and the lining of the mouth. However, depending on where Mary is in her life plan and whether or not she has other illnesses may still make her choose all treatments that can offer even a small improvement in her chances.

Figure 81 shows the number of lives potentially saved (shown in orange) if we treated 100 patients like Angela or 100 like Mary. We have to treat 100 women with chemotherapy for the potential benefit of ten in Angela's situation and only two in Mary's situation. If I were Angela, I would certainly be having chemotherapy because the survival rates look a lot better with it. If I were Mary on the other hand I would probably lean towards no additional treatment or giving hormonal treatment a try.

The main point here is to try to understand the statistics in your own situation and weigh up all the benefits and risks. Also remember that you can always change your mind after a few courses of treatment if you can't cope with the side effects. For example, if Mary decides that she wants to give chemotherapy a go and copes very well, then she may as well complete at least four courses. If, on the other hand, the drugs don't agree with her, then maybe she should stop, given that the benefit is small. In Angela's case, however, I think the pain is really worth the potential 10 percentage point gain.

Angela

No Chemotherapy

10-year survival (green) if chemotherapy is not used: 60%

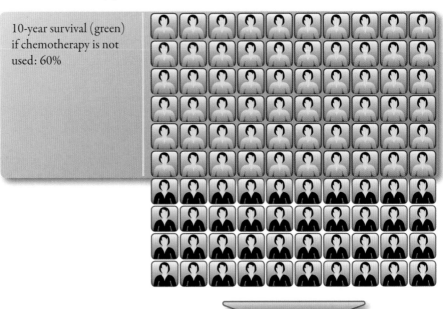

Angela

Chemotherapy

Additional benefit from chemotherapy on 10-year survival rate (orange): 10%

10-year survival if chemotherapy is used (green and orange): 70%

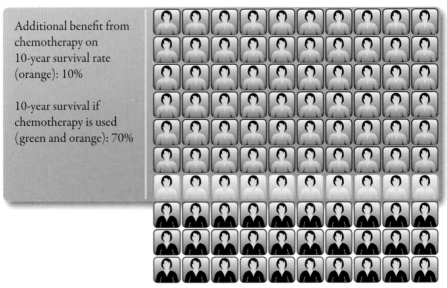

Figure 81a: Angela has a higher risk of dying from breast cancer but also a larger benefit from chemotherapy. Women in orange show additional lives saved from chemotherapy.

Mary

No Chemotherapy

10-year survival rate (green) if chemotherapy is not used: 92%

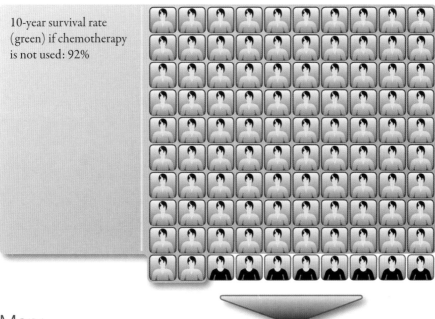

Mary

Chemotherapy

Additional benefit from chemotherapy on 10-year survival rate (orange): 2%

10-year survival if chemotherapy is used (green and orange): 94%

Figure 81b: Mary has a lower risk of dying from breast cancer and a smaller benefit from chemotherapy. Women in orange show additional lives saved from chemotherapy.

Maria's Story

Maria was a 63-year-old Greek woman who came to see me for advice about chemotherapy. Her glands were not involved. Her tumor was hormone sensitive.

She didn't speak English very well, but with my broken Greek, I was able to get her through some of the concepts.

I told her that the absolute benefit from chemotherapy was around one percent and the absolute benefit from Tamoxifen was also around one to two percent. She went and saw another oncologist, who told her that he could give her a "30 percent improvement" from chemotherapy. He was talking about a 30 percent reduction in the risk.

This statistic, when quoted to patients, is very misleading. Of course she went with the other practitioner, who gave her a better prognosis than I could, by presenting the statistics in a more "inflated" way.

Beware the oncologist who just talks about "relapse" or "recurrence," which is also misleading because it over-inflates the chance of your cancer coming back. Relapse statistics include all sorts of "events" that cannot be controlled by chemotherapy, such as getting breast cancer on the other side (which is not reduced by chemotherapy), dying in a car accident or from another cause, and getting a cancer totally unrelated to breast cancer.

In summary:

- Take control

- Understand the statistics

- Question the statistics

- Understand what your baseline cure rate is without chemotherapy or hormonal treatment

- Understand what your chances of dying of other causes or old age are—if, for example, your chance of dying from other causes is high or much higher than dying from breast cancer (Table 12)

- Be careful of the oncologist who quotes odds ratios or odds reductions or reductions in the risk of relapse, as they may be making chemotherapy sound better than it is and may lead you into a decision that's not absolutely necessary

- For patients who are older with hormone-positive tumors, hormone tablets such as tamoxifen and aromatase inhibitors may provide most of the benefit

- For younger women who are hormone sensitive, chemotherapy alone is probably not enough, and some sort of hormonal manipulation will be necessary.

As mentioned earlier, the fabulous calculator at Adjuvantonline.com has really helped specialists estimate prognosis. This has been a real bonus for both patients and doctors, and Peter Ravdin, the leader in this field, has added a great deal of information to the website so that busy doctors can keep up with the latest statistics.

What's my chance of dying of something else?

Most chemotherapy research trials have enrolled women who are in general fit for their age. The Adjuvant! Online calculator allows an adjustment if you are less fit than average.

When your doctor considers and works out whether or not to give you chemotherapy, he or she also has to take into account your chance of dying of something else or of old age.

Basically, the older you are, the more reluctant I would be to give you chemotherapy, particularly if you have a lot of other illnesses.

Chemotherapy doesn't work as well as you get older and often has more side effects. If your tumor is ER-positive, hormonal treatment is a better approach. Table 12 shows the latest US life expectancy statistics (Arias 2006).

If you are older and fit, remember that you may still have a lot of years ahead of you.

Seventy is not that old—you have

Age	Life Expectancy (All Races)
0	80
10	71
20	61
30	51
35	46
40	42
45	37
50	32
55	28
60	24
65	20
70	16
75	13
80	10
85	7
90	5
95	4
100	3

Table 12: Average life expectancy if you didn't get breast cancer

another 16 years on average to live, and you may indeed live to be 100!

So the trick is not to be over-treated or under-treated. I'm not saying you should never get chemotherapy, but neither should you be talked out of having breast conservation or an immediate reconstruction if you're having a mastectomy.

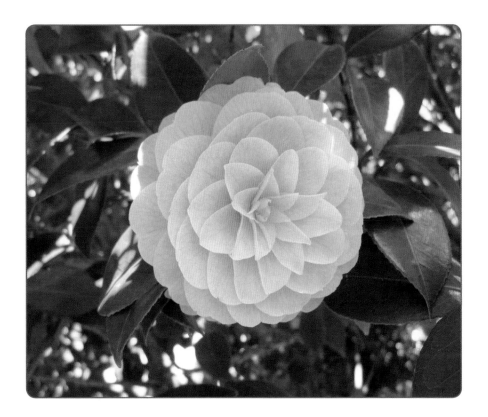

CONTROL POINT #15 – WHAT DO THE STATISTICS REALLY MEAN?

WARNING

Be careful of the oncologist who quotes only "relapse" statistics, as they may be making the benefit from chemotherapy sound better than it really is.

TIP

First, understand what your baseline survival rate is without chemotherapy or hormonal treatment. Also understand what your chances of dying of other causes or old age are to put your risk from breast cancer into perspective.

REMEMBER

Statistics are only a guide to your prognosis at the point of diagnosis. Your chances improve over time, particularly after you reach five years post-diagnosis.

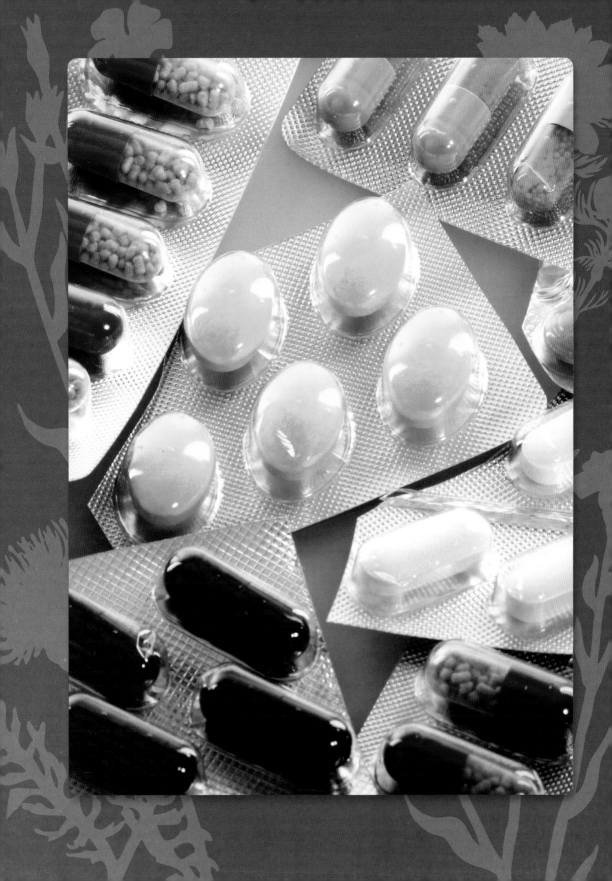

Control Point 16

Do I Need Hormonal Treatment?

Control Point #16

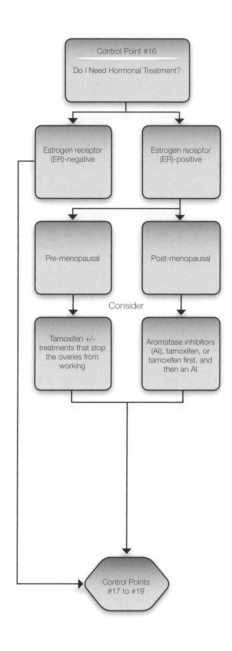

Control Point #16

Do I Need Hormonal Treatment?

Estrogen receptor (ER)-negative

Estrogen receptor (ER)-positive

Pre-menopausal

Post-menopausal

Consider

Tamoxifen +/- treatments that stop the ovaries from working

Aromatase inhibitors (AI), tamoxifen, or tamoxifen first, and then an AI

Control Points #17 to #19

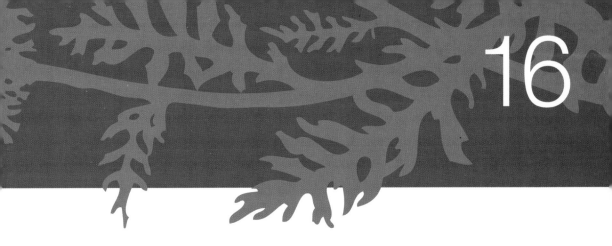

Do I Need Hormonal Treatment?

Yet another garden analogy

Let's get back to my garden basics for a moment. Sometimes when we find a weed under the rose bush, and that weed also involves the next garden patch, we really need to think about whether some seeds could already have spread or been blown by the wind to other parts of the garden (Figure 80).

I don't mean seeds that have already grown into weeds that we can see, but rather seeds we can't see but that could become dangerous weeds in the future. The next two chapters deal with whether or not we need to use "weed killer" on the other parts of the garden after removing the weed under the rose bush. In other words, do we need to give some precautionary chemotherapy or hormonal treatment as a form of "weed killer" just in case your cancer has thrown off some seeds via your blood stream to other parts of your body?

Hopefully, your breast cancer has not spread beyond your breast or glands, but sometimes we need to treat the rest of your body just in case. As mentioned earlier, this depends on many factors, but is considered particularly if your glands are involved or if your cancer is large, high grade, or not responsive to estrogen (ER-negative).

This additional or "adjuvant" treatment is, in some ways, a bit of extra insurance. Taking hormonal treatments is a softer option with fewer side effects than chemotherapy and a good approach if we can get away with it. It's perhaps more like using a spray-on attachment for your hose to treat the other parts of the garden away from the rose bush. Having chemotherapy is more like using a toxic, professional weed-killer service. You can imagine this more intensive weed killer would cost more, work better and potentially cause some harm to other normal plants in the garden.

Sound scientific evidence has shown that there is a greater chance of killing off cancer cells when they are small and invisible to the naked eye, before they become dangerous spots or breast cancer. In this chapter, I will explain how estrogen that is produced in your body, even after you go through menopause, can act as a "fertilizer" and feed ER-positive breast cancer cells that may already have spread to other parts of the body. Reducing the level of estrogen or blocking it from working can help destroy these cancer cells.

How estrogen is made in the body

Estrogen is a hormone produced by the ovaries until you reach menopause, and produced in small quantities by the adrenal glands, fat, and muscle tissue before and after you've gone through menopause.

Figure 82 shows some of the hormones produced by the different glands in your body before or after menopause. In the brain, an area just above the pituitary gland (called the hypothalamus) stimulates the pituitary with a compound called "luteinizing hormone releasing hormone" (LHRH), which then produces pituitary hormones called "follicle-stimulating hormone" (FSH) and "luteinizing hormone" (LH) which stimulate the ovaries and the pituitary hormone adrenocorticotropic hormone (ACTH), which stimulates the adrenal glands. In short, these stimulate the ovaries to produce "female-type" hormones called estrogen and progesterone, and the adrenal gland (mainly an issue in women who have gone through the menopause) to convert a "male-type" hormone called androgen to estrogen in very small amounts using an enzyme called aromatase. Estrogen, FSH and LH levels can be measured in your blood to work out if you have gone through the menopause.

Understanding the estrogen receptor

There are a few different ways in which we can block the effect of estrogen or lower estrogen levels. Even though we call the treatment "hormonal therapy" or "hormone therapy," we really mean "anti-hormone" therapy, because what we are trying to do is to reduce the level of estrogen in your body to stop it from stimulating the estrogen receptor. That's why I call it "hormonal treatment" so it's not confused with "HRT" (hormone replacement therapy) or "HT" (hormone therapy) when extra estrogen is taken after the menopause.

I sometimes compare this estrogen pathway to how a television works. The very large TV antenna at, for example, ABC TV, is like your pituitary gland, which sends signals to two smaller repeater antennas (the ovary and the adrenal gland) that send out the signal to your home.

The TV aerial on the roof of your house is like the estrogen receptor, and the TV in your living area is like the cancer cell. Houses with antennas are a bit like ER-positive breast cancer. If they get the signal, the TV works when you press the "power" switch. Similarly, ER-positive breast cancer can be turned on by the estrogen that is normally made by your body.

An ER-negative breast cancer is like the houses getting cable TV with no antenna (Figure 83). We need compounds other than hormones to treat these cancers via a different route. The aim of hormonal treatment is to "starve" breast cancer cells of the hormone (estrogen) that may stimulate them to grow. Long-term research has shown that stopping estrogen from stimulating any leftover hormone-sensitive cells lowers the risk of cancer coming back not only elsewhere in the body, but also in the treated breast (even after a mastectomy) and the other breast.

There are two broad hormonal approaches that can be used on this complex hormonal pathway: drugs that block the effect of estrogen on cancer cells, called anti-estrogens; and removing or "turning off" the ovaries.

Anti-estrogen medicines do not decrease estrogen levels. Instead, they prevent estrogen from causing the breast cancer cells to grow, by blocking the estrogen receptor that may be present on your breast cancer cell.

These work a bit like putting a lead shield around the TV antenna on your roof. The signal from the main transmission antenna is still there, but it can't make contact with your TV antenna, so your TV stops working.

Drugs or treatments that lower estrogen levels in the body include the aromatase inhibitors (such as anastrozole [Arimidex] or letrozole [Femara] or exemestane [Aromasin]), the LHRH agonists such as **goserelin [Zoladex]**, and stopping the ovaries from working by either removing them or (less commonly) giving them radiation (Figure 82).

Removing or stopping the ovaries from working is like knocking out one of the repeater antennas receiving the ABC signal, which stops your TV from working.

BEFORE THE MENOPAUSE

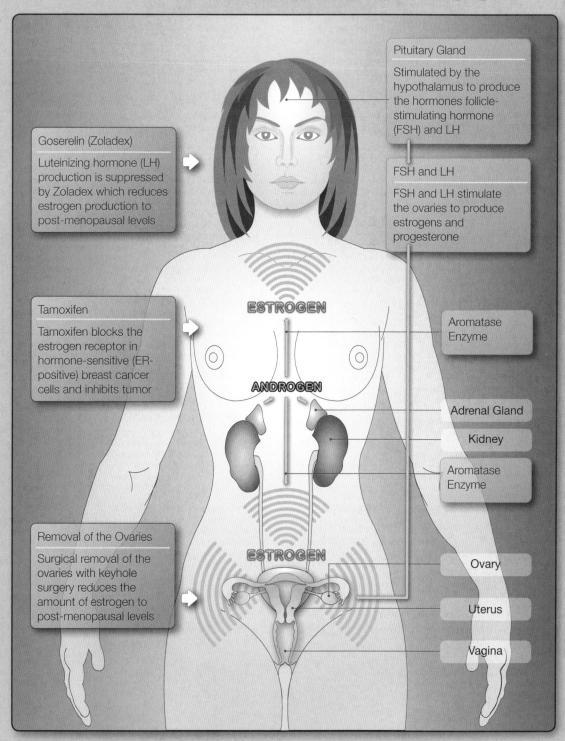

Goserelin (Zoladex)

Luteinizing hormone (LH) production is suppressed by Zoladex which reduces estrogen production to post-menopausal levels

Pituitary Gland

Stimulated by the hypothalamus to produce the hormones follicle-stimulating hormone (FSH) and LH

FSH and LH

FSH and LH stimulate the ovaries to produce estrogens and progesterone

Tamoxifen

Tamoxifen blocks the estrogen receptor in hormone-sensitive (ER-positive) breast cancer cells and inhibits tumor

Removal of the Ovaries

Surgical removal of the ovaries with keyhole surgery reduces the amount of estrogen to post-menopausal levels

ESTROGEN

ANDROGEN

ESTROGEN

Aromatase Enzyme

Adrenal Gland

Kidney

Aromatase Enzyme

Ovary

Uterus

Vagina

Figure 82a: How estrogen is made in your body before the menopause.

AFTER THE MENOPAUSE

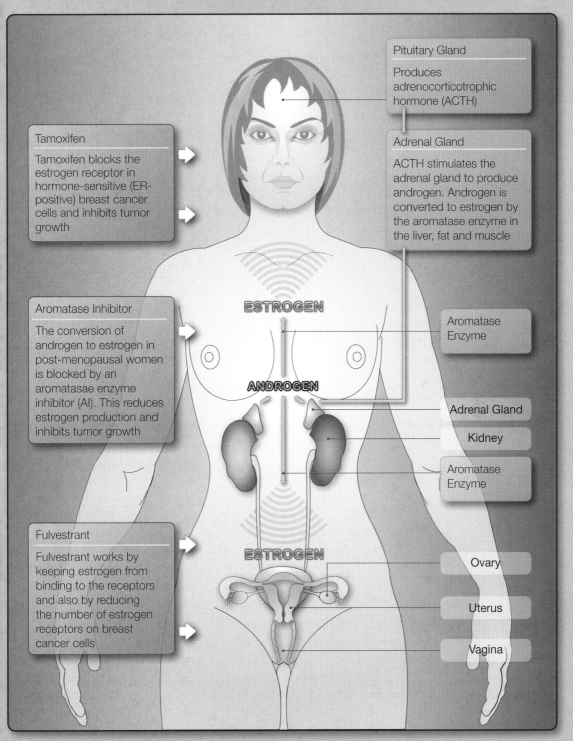

Pituitary Gland

Produces adrenocorticotrophic hormone (ACTH)

Tamoxifen

Tamoxifen blocks the estrogen receptor in hormone-sensitive (ER-positive) breast cancer cells and inhibits tumor growth

Adrenal Gland

ACTH stimulates the adrenal gland to produce androgen. Androgen is converted to estrogen by the aromatase enzyme in the liver, fat and muscle

ESTROGEN

Aromatase Inhibitor

The conversion of androgen to estrogen in post-menopausal women is blocked by an aromatasae enzyme inhibitor (AI). This reduces estrogen production and inhibits tumor growth

Aromatase Enzyme

ANDROGEN

Adrenal Gland

Kidney

Aromatase Enzyme

Fulvestrant

Fulvestrant works by keeping estrogen from binding to the receptors and also by reducing the number of estrogen receptors on breast cancer cells

ESTROGEN

Ovary

Uterus

Vagina

Figure 82b: How estrogen is made in your body after the menopause.

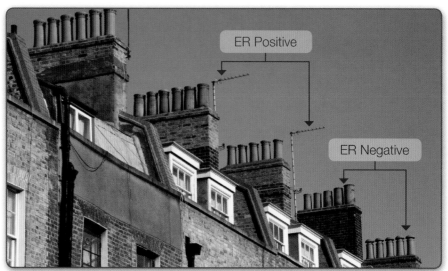

Figure 83: The television antenna system is a bit like the estrogen pathway in your body—stopping estrogen from reaching an ER-positive cancer cell is like putting a lead shield around the antenna outside your house. The TV inside now doesn't work.

Anti-estrogen drugs: tamoxifen

Tamoxifen has been used for over 30 years and is a true and tested drug in the treatment of breast cancer. Tamoxifen is also known as a **selective estrogen receptor modulator (SERM)** because it acts like estrogen on some tissues but blocks the effect of estrogen on other tissues. Tamoxifen (Nolvadex) and raloxifene (Evista) are two examples of SERMs.

Estrogen (shown in orange in Figure 84) is used by the cell if it finds a receptor on the cell's surface. The estrogen receptor complex activates the cancer cells' genetic code or "DNA" and can cause it to grow. Tamoxifen (shown in purple in Figure 84) blocks the receptors in breast tissue and stops estrogen from working. Basically, tamoxifen works by "pretending" it is estrogen and binding to the estrogen receptor. Because it is a weak estrogen, it can sometimes stimulate estrogen receptors in other parts of the body, such as your womb, and in very rare circumstances cause unwanted side effects such as polyps or even cancer of the womb.

Tamoxifen is broken down into its active form in the liver by an enzyme called CYP2D6, which is produced by a gene called 2D6. This enzyme is necessary for the body to metabolize a number of drugs, including tamoxifen. It's estimated that about one in ten women with breast cancer have a gene variant that keeps their bodies from properly metabolizing tamoxifen. Some oncologists test their patients for the CYP2D6 enzyme before starting tamoxifen, but this has not become routine practice as of yet (Ferraldeschi 2010).

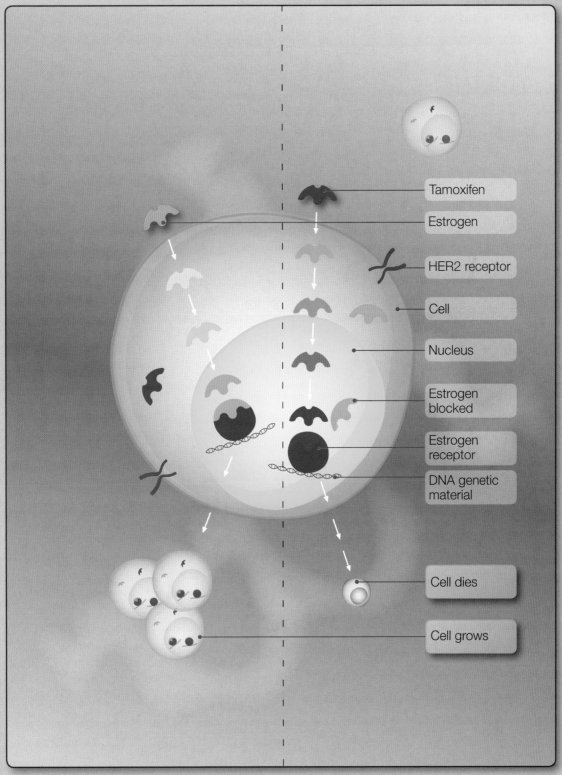

Tamoxifen

Estrogen

HER2 receptor

Cell

Nucleus

Estrogen blocked

Estrogen receptor

DNA genetic material

Cell dies

Cell grows

Figure 84: The ER-positive breast cancer cell grows if fed with estrogen (orange), or shrinks and dies from estrogen being blocked by tamoxifen (purple).

How is tamoxifen taken, and for how long?

Tamoxifen is taken by mouth. The usual dose is 20 mg a day, and it's usually started after surgery or after the completion of radiation treatment (Figure 86, strategy A, H, I or T). If you have chemotherapy after surgery, your treatment with tamoxifen will start once you have finished the chemotherapy. Research has shown that giving the two treatments together not only reduces the beneficial effect of each compound, but it also increases the chance of complications such as a blood clot. It is also thought that giving tamoxifen at the same time as radiation reduces its beneficial effect.

You can take tamoxifen with or without food, at any time during the day, but you should take it at the same time each day. If you like to take tablets in the morning ("to get them out of the way for the day") just add them to any other medications you may be taking. If you prefer to take tamoxifen at bedtime, that's fine as well.

You should not become pregnant or breastfeed while taking tamoxifen, or for two to three months after stopping. While tamoxifen can stop your periods and you may feel as if you've gone through menopause, you may still be fertile. You should use some form of contraception other than the oral contraceptive pill, like barrier contraception (such as condoms or a diaphragm with spermicide) or intrauterine devices (IUDs), because the pill may alter the effects of the tamoxifen (see Control Point #18 – Will Treatment Affect My Periods, Fertility, or Sex Life?).

Currently, the recommended length for tamoxifen therapy is five years. There have been a couple of studies showing that taking tamoxifen for ten years did not have any additional benefit to taking it over five years, and instead increased the risk of getting cancer of the womb (endometrium).

A recent trial called "ATLAS," or Adjuvant Tamoxifen — Longer Against Shorter, was presented at the 30th Annual San Antonio Breast Cancer Symposium in December 2007. It involved 11,500 patients from more than 400 hospitals. This trial compared women taking five years of tamoxifen with longer periods, up to ten years. The statistics are a little complicated, but the trial suggested that longer periods of tamoxifen may not be as bad as we think. For example, if you have had a hysterectomy (and therefore there is no risk of **endometrial cancer** (cancer of the womb), then in some situations if your risk of cancer coming back is still thought to be on the high side and you can't tolerate or afford aromatase inhibitors (see below), continuing tamoxifen may be a reasonable alternative. We are still awaiting the final published results of this study.

What are the benefits of tamoxifen?

Tamoxifen treatment can reduce the chance of breast cancer returning after breast surgery if you have a cancer that is estrogen receptor-positive. It acts against the effects of estrogen in the breast, but as mentioned, it may act like estrogen in other tissues, so it may also provide some of the beneficial effects of estrogen; some studies have found that it reduces the risk of heart disease by lowering cholesterol and may also reduce the chance of **osteoporosis**.

Tamoxifen may improve cure rates by a few percentage points (one to ten percent) and reduce the risk of breast cancer in the opposite breast from 1 in 200 each year to 1 in 300 to 400. It also reduces the chance of cancer coming back locally in the breast after breast conservation, and in the chest wall and lymph glands after a mastectomy. As explained in Control Point #15 – What Do The Statistics Really Mean? the benefit of tamoxifen may be quite small if you have a tiny cancer that hasn't spread to any lymph glands.

What are the side effects of tamoxifen?

Many women don't experience any side effects at all. The most common side effects are minor, and they usually lessen as treatment continues and cease when treatment stops. Tamoxifen does not cause menopause, but its side effects are similar and can include:

- Hot flashes (called "flushes" in the UK, Australia, and elsewhere) or sweats

- Irregular menstrual periods (if you have not gone through menopause)

- Cessation of your menstruation

- Vaginal irritation, dryness, or discharge

- Fluid retention and weight gain. We don't really know if weight gain is due to the tamoxifen or just because people are getting older and may be less active. In one study where tamoxifen or a sugar tablet (placebo) was given to women who only had a family history of breast cancer, to see if it could prevent breast cancer, both groups of women gained weight.

Uncommon side effects may include light-headedness, thinning hair, aches and pains in the joints, dizziness, headache, and tiredness. These usually get better after taking tamoxifen for a few weeks. Taking a half dose of tamoxifen (10 mg per day) for about four weeks and then going up to the full dose may help your body get used to these side effects. An allergic type rash is very rare, as is nausea. Some women (e.g. who are in a choir or sing) may experience a slight deepening of their voice, as can occur naturally after menopause.

A rare complication (less than 1-in-100 chance at ten years) is the development of cancer of the uterus (womb), also known as endometrial or uterine cancer. The additional risk of cancer of the uterus is about 1 per 1,000 women per year taking tamoxifen. So if you take tamoxifen for five years, the additional risk is 5 in 1,000, or 1 in 200. In other words, the risk is real but very low. Any abnormal vaginal bleeding should be reported to your doctor, who will decide whether further investigation is needed. Spotting can occur in women who have not gone through the menopause.

A routine gynecological check is advised before you start tamoxifen. There does not appear to be any benefit to having routine pelvic scans such as ultrasound (they are usually abnormal while on tamoxifen and serve no real purpose) for women who are taking tamoxifen. An annual pelvic check and Pap smear is a good idea when you are on tamoxifen and as part of your general health.

The risk of thrombosis (a blood clot) or embolism (a blood clot that travels) is the same as the risk of blood clots for women on the birth control pill or hormone replacement therapy. Report any sign of leg swelling or pain to your doctor. I normally recommend stopping tamoxifen for about one week before you travel if you're going to be immobile for long periods of time (such as long flights, car trips, or surgery) to try to prevent blood clots also known such as the "economy class syndrome" or deep venous thrombosis (DVT).

Very rarely, tamoxifen can result in depression or mood swings. If this occurs, it may worthwhile you changing from tamoxifen to something else. Also, fine facial hair may become more prominent on tamoxifen. The risk of **cataract** may increase slightly for women taking tamoxifen, although this occurs normally as people age regardless. Other eye problems, such as corneal scarring or retinal changes, have been reported in a few patients.

A rare form of inflammation of the back of the eye can be serious. Stop tamoxifen immediately and see an eye doctor as soon as possible if you are having visual disturbances.

I have seen two patients in the past 25 years or so whose platelet counts have dropped. Platelets are cells in the blood that help with blood clotting. If you get unexplained bruising, stop the medication and get an urgent **blood count**. I have also seen one patient with a drop in her white cells (the cells that fight infection), but not to dangerous levels. In all these patients, their blood counts returned to normal after they stopped the tamoxifen.

Can tamoxifen be used with other medications?

Tamoxifen can interact with warfarin (a drug used to prevent blood clotting), and you should remind your doctor if you're taking it because your blood levels may need closer monitoring for a while. Do not take other hormone treatments if you're taking tamoxifen, but continue to take any other drugs that your doctor has prescribed.

Other hormone receptor blocking agents

Toremifene (Fareston) is another anti-estrogen drug closely related to tamoxifen. It may be an option for women who have gone through the menopause, but government restrictions often restrict this to women with breast cancer that has spread. It has a similar range of side effects to tamoxifen, but is said to have a lower incidence of cancer of the womb.

Fulvestrant (Faslodex) is a newer drug that reduces the number of estrogen receptors. It is effective for women after menopause, even if their breast cancer is no longer responding to tamoxifen. Hot flashes, mild nausea, and fatigue are the major side effects of fulvestrant. It works by keeping estrogen from binding to the receptors and also by reducing the number of estrogen receptors on breast cancer cells. It may help when other treatment has failed; in clinical trials, fulvestrant was found to be effective when tamoxifen no longer worked. Faslodex is given every four weeks directly into the muscle. For women whose cancer has spread, fulvestrant is often funded by insurance companies or, in some countries, the government.

Raloxifene (Evista) is another drug that has been shown to reduce the incidence of breast cancer and the chance of breast cancer developing in women with a family history, but as yet, there are no studies proving that it works once you have breast cancer. It is also known as a "selective estrogen receptor modulator" (SERM), One small study tested high-dose raloxifene on 22 women whose cancer had come back, but the trial had to be stopped because of low response rates. Four of the 22 women had some response, but the disease did not go away completely in any woman (Gradishar 2000). We are not currently recommending raloxifene for women with breast cancer, even for the treatment of osteoporosis. It has been approved in the US and Australia for reducing future breast cancer developmet in post-menopausal women who have a strong family history of breast cancer and for women with certain pre-cancerous changes on a biopsy (Visanathan 2009).

Drugs that lower estrogen levels: aromatase inhibitors

Aromatase inhibitors (AIs) stop the small amounts of estrogen being produced in your body after you have reached the menopause. Three drugs in this class are available for treatment of breast cancer: anastrozole (Arimidex), letrozole (Femara), and exemestane (Aromasin).

These drugs work by blocking an enzyme (aromatase) that helps make estrogen in post-menopausal women by helping to convert it from androgen produced in places like the adrenal gland (see Figure 82b). They cannot stop the ovaries of pre-menopausal women from making estrogen because there is too much circulating estrogen for them to work.

For this reason, they are only effective in post-menopausal women. For pre-menopausal women, tamoxifen remains the best drug to use. Aromatase inhibitors can work in younger women who become post-menopausal after chemotherapy (see Control Point #18 – Will Treatment Affect My Periods, Fertility, or Sex Life?). It can also work in women who have had their ovarian function stopped deliberately by surgical removal or drugs such as goserelin, which is branded as Zoladex (see below). If you are taking an aromatase inhibitor and you have a period, talk to your oncologist as soon as possible.

The aromatase inhibitors have been compared with tamoxifen as adjuvant hormonal treatment in several clinical trials. They have somewhat different side effects than tamoxifen because they don't cause cancer of the uterus and very rarely cause blood clots. They can, however, slightly increase the chances of osteoporosis and bone fractures because they remove all estrogen from a post-menopausal woman. They also cause hot flashes and sometimes joint and muscle pain.

How is an aromatase inhibitor taken and for how long?

AIs come as pills that you take once a day. It is best to take them at the same time every day. If you miss a dose, you don't need to take an extra dose the next day. The level of the drug in your body will remain high enough from the previous day.

After local therapies such as surgery or radiation therapy, if you have not been given tamoxifen, you will usually take an AI for five years. If you have been given tamoxifen, you will take it for two to three years, and then you will probably switch to an AI for two to three years (for a total of five years of therapy). One study has shown that after five years of tamoxifen, five years of Femara is helpful. Nobody really knows the right duration, or whether or not everybody should get a total of ten years of treatment, or even longer, and clinical trials are ongoing to work this out. The Adjuvant! Online calculator works out how much better your chances are with Femara after taking tamoxifen for five years. In general, if your prognosis was pretty good at the start (a node-negative, small cancer) the extra benefits are small. If you had node-positive disease or a larger tumor, then it's probably worthwhile giving aromatase inhibitors a try.

What are the benefits of an aromatase inhibitor?

The aromatase inhibitors are slightly more effective than tamoxifen alone in preventing breast cancer from coming back for post-menopausal women. However, it's not all that clear cut, and one size doesn't fit all. If your breast cancer has been detected early with negative nodes, or if you or your mother have a history of significant osteoporosis, then you still may be better off having tamoxifen only. If your cancer is more serious (say a higher-grade cancer, or larger than 20 mm, or with positive nodes), then an aromatase inhibitor is slightly better.

I prefer the approach of giving tamoxifen for two to three years (which may strengthen the bones) and then switching to an AI if you're around 50 and we're not sure if you've gone through menopause, particularly because your periods may only have stopped temporarily after chemotherapy.

The problem is that if you haven't gone through menopause, an AI can stimulate ovulation (eggs produced by the ovaries), and there have been one or two cases of unexpected pregnancies (Smith 2006).

When is an aromatase inhibitor prescribed?

There have been several types of clinical trials comparing different combinations of tamoxifen and AIs (Figure 85). These trials have tested whether giving an AI instead of tamoxifen or using various combinations of tamoxifen and an AI were better than the standard treatment of five years of tamoxifen.

The first type of clinical trial examined a direct, head-to-head comparison of tamoxifen versus an AI for five years for women who have gone through the menopause, and the AI was slightly better.

The second trial type examined a comparison of five years of tamoxifen with two to three years of tamoxifen and then an AI for a total of five years of treatment, and again, women who received an AI did slightly better.

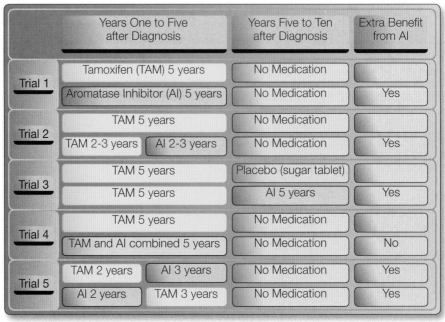

	Years One to Five after Diagnosis		Years Five to Ten after Diagnosis	Extra Benefit from AI
Trial 1	Tamoxifen (TAM) 5 years		No Medication	
	Aromatase Inhibitor (AI) 5 years		No Medication	Yes
Trial 2	TAM 5 years		No Medication	
	TAM 2-3 years	AI 2-3 years	No Medication	Yes
Trial 3	TAM 5 years		Placebo (sugar tablet)	
	TAM 5 years		AI 5 years	Yes
Trial 4	TAM 5 years		No Medication	
	TAM and AI combined 5 years		No Medication	No
Trial 5	TAM 2 years	AI 3 years	No Medication	Yes
	AI 2 years	TAM 3 years	No Medication	Yes

Figure 85: Trials of tamoxifen versus aromatase inhibitors—sequence and duration.

The third trial type compared giving a sugar tablet (placebo) or an AI for a further five years after five years of tamoxifen, and again there was a slight extra benefit in taking an AI. The fourth trial type combined tamoxifen and an AI, and for some reason, this group of patients did worse than those who took tamoxifen alone. The fifth type of trial compared whether starting tamoxifen or an AI for the first two years and then switching to the second drug for the next three years made any difference.

Nearly all studies have found that AIs simply increase the time it takes for cancer to come back, but the overall cure (survival) rates are the same whether or not patients took tamoxifen first or an AI first. One study suggests a small survival benefit from taking two to three years of tamoxifen and then switching over to an AI. What this means is that you don't have to get anxious if you can't tolerate an AI for some reason. In 2009, an international panel of experts in St Gallen suggested that an AI should be considered standard treatment, particularly if the risk of breast cancer coming back was high (Goldhirsch 2009).

Some doctors have stopped using tamoxifen completely for women who have gone through menopause, and this is reasonable if there are no contraindications. In terms of which one to use—Arimidex, Femara, or Aromasin—they're probably all about the same, but different countries have different rules. One oncologist I work with tells me he flips a coin outside the consult room to decide! In general, if your prognosis is not that bad or your bones are bad, I use tamoxifen first; if the prognosis is worse and your bones are good, I use an AI. As mentioned above, another reason to use tamoxifen is if you're not really sure if you've gone through menopause, particularly if you're in your late forties or very early fifties. Even if your periods have stopped after chemotherapy, it's best to see if they come back over the next year or to check your blood hormone levels a few times over the next six to 12 months to be certain that your ovaries have stopped working and you are definitely post-menopausal.

What are the side effects of an aromatase inhibitor?

Although many women do not experience any side effects from aromatase inhibitors, muscle aches and pains can occur in up to one in three women. Usually, they are not severe. Estrogen helps with lubrication of the joints and many women have increasing joint stiffness as they go through the natural menopause. Although all hormonal treatments of breast cancer can cause joint stiffness it is more common with aromatase inhibitors. These can improve as you keep taking the drug. I have seen only one patient who had to resort to a walking stick because of her pain, so I insisted she take tamoxifen instead. Treatment options for joint pains are discussed in Control Point #18. Hot flashes can occur but are usually slightly less frequent than those caused by tamoxifen (about 25–30 percent).

One study found that sexual side effects were far worse on AIs than on tamoxifen. They can reduce sex drive and can rarely change your orgasm or make it disappear altogether. Use a lubricant rather than vaginal estrogen if you're having problems with painful intercourse. Because aromatase inhibitors block the very small amounts of estrogen in your body after menopause, and vaginal estrogen is absorbed slightly through the vaginal wall, the two, at least theoretically, don't really work well together (Kendall 2006).

Less common side effects may include nausea, vomiting, loss of appetite, or diarrhea. These symptoms tend to be mild and temporary and can usually be helped by taking your medication with food. If the symptoms don't improve, talk to your doctor. Like tamoxifen, slight changes in voice can also occur.

Insomnia is also a possibility while on AIs. I have stopped Arimidex on two occasions because of this particularly disruptive side effect. Fatigue is possible as well. Though there are many potential causes of fatigue, particularly chemotherapy, AIs can be the culprit for some patients. Other less common side effects may include headache, skin rash, or sleepiness. These are usually temporary and should wear off after a short time. One study found no difference in memory function between women taking a sugar pill and women with a strong family history of breast cancer taking Arimidex to prevent breast cancer (Jenkins 2008).

Vaginal bleeding is a rare side effect of aromatase inhibitors. This can happen in the first few weeks after starting the treatment. If it persists, consult your doctor to arrange a check. Cancer of the womb is not increased with aromatase inhibitors.

Bone thinning or osteoporosis is a side effect of AIs and is discussed in detail below. If you already have thinning of the bones, you may be better off starting with tamoxifen and then switching to an AI. Recent studies have found that drugs such as **bisphosphonates** reduce the risk of osteoporosis for women taking AIs and are another alternative that allows such women to keep using them. Also, some pharmaceutical companies are providing free access to these drugs.

Bisphosphonates can be given as tablets or as a once- or twice-yearly injection. One study found that zoledronic acid (Zometa) given in a dose of 4 mg through an intravenous drip every six months prevented thinning of the bones for patients who were taking an AI or tamoxifen with goserelin (Zoladex). These studies also suggested that Zometa may help delay the recurrence of breast cancer (Gnant 2008, 2009). A very rare complication from bisphosphonates is osteonecrosis of the jaw where part of the jaw bone fails to heal after surgery. A check by a dental surgeon before commencing bisphonotaes is often recommended (Vahtsevanos 2009).

Can an aromatase inhibitor be used with other medications?

Drugs containing estrogen, such as HRT or the contraceptive pill, should not be taken with aromatase inhibitors because they stop it from working effectively. As mentioned above, although we can't be sure about this, it's probably best to avoid vaginal estrogen while you are taking an aromatase inhibitor. If you're on warfarin for blood clots, let your doctor know to keep a close check on your blood tests, as sometimes your warfarin levels will need adjusting.

Understanding osteoporosis

Osteoporosis, or bone thinning, makes your bones more fragile and susceptible to fracture. One study found that when you take an aromatase inhibitor as your hormonal treatment, there is a 50 percent chance of thinning of the bones (**osteopenia**) and a 10 percent chance of osteoporosis.

One large international study called "ATAC," or "Arimidex, Tamoxifen Alone or in Combination," compared a total of five years of tamoxifen to five years of Arimidex (Trial Type 1 in Figure 85), and found that fractures were slightly higher for Arimidex. The incidence of fractures was 11 percent for Arimidex and 8 percent for tamoxifen after nearly six years of follow-up (Chien 2006).

The Breast International Group (BIG) studied this question in the "BIG 1-98" trial and also found that fractures were slightly higher for patients taking an AI. This trial, an example of Trial Type 5 in Figure 85), compared three years of Femara (letrozole) after two years of tamoxifen or vice versa and found that, after about two years of follow-up, the incidence of fractures was 6 percent for women taking letrozole and 4 percent for women who only took tamoxifen (Chien 2006).

It's a good idea to check your blood vitamin D level before you start your treatment, as low vitamin D levels are common. This is mainly because we're not getting enough sun exposure for our bodies to make vitamin D or eating enough foods that are good sources of vitamin D. The term "vitamin D" encompasses two molecules: vitamin D3 formed in the skin through the action of sunlight or obtained from animal sources in the diet; and vitamin D2, a plant source of vitamin D also available through the diet. Vitamin D helps to regulate the absorption of calcium through the intestine, which is required to strengthen our bones.

Recent evidence suggests that having a low vitamin D level may increase the risk of breast cancer coming back, but more research is required to confirm this finding (Goodwin 2008). Small amounts of sun exposure every day are important for increasing your vitamin D levels naturally. Just ten minutes in the sun on most days of the week in summer, 15 to 20 minutes in spring and autumn, or 30 minutes in winter, outside peak UV times (10 am–2 pm, or 11 am–3 pm daylight savings time), will usually give you enough vitamin D (NSW Cancer Council 2008).

The closer you live to the equator, the shorter the duration of sun exposure is required. For those who live in far northern or southern latitudes, the UV level in the winter months is inadequate for any vitamin D to be produced by the body, so fortified foods or supplements may be required . . . or an annual tropical holiday! Vitamin D deficiency is more common if your body is fully covered with an abaya and hijab or if you have dark skin.

A baseline measurement of **bone mineral density** should be obtained before you start your AI treatment. The World Health Organization (WHO) has recognized a dual-energy X-ray absorptiometry (DEXA) scan as the most convenient, accurate and reproducible method to measure bone mineral density. Bone mineral density is a measurement of the level of minerals (mainly calcium) in the bones, which is an indication of their strength. WHO have classified this as a "T-score", which is a measurement of your bone density compared with that of a young, healthy adult woman (Table 13).

T–score	Definition
More than 1.0	Normal
Between −1.0 and −2.5	Osteopenia
Less than −2.5	Osteoporosis
Less than −2.5 and breaks due to fragile bones	Severe osteoporosis

Table 13: World Health Organization score for bone health

As well as your vitamin D levels, serum calcium and magnesium levels should also be checked before starting bisphosphonate therapy, and parathyroid hormone testing should be considered. Some doctors order a urine test that measures chemicals which can show whether or not there is high bone turnover or loss. You may need to be referred to an endocrinologist if you have established osteoporosis. Based on the National Osteoporosis Foundation guidelines, women with no risk factors for osteoporosis should begin bisphosphonate therapy if their T-score is −2.0 or below.

Women with risk factors should begin therapy to help slow or reverse their bone loss if their T-score is −1.5 or below. Risk factors for osteoporosis include age over 65, being thin or short, a previous history of a fracture as an adult, a family history of osteoporosis, chronic steroid use, inadequate weight-bearing physical activity, being white or Asian, consuming excessive caffeine from cola or coffee, smoking cigarettes, drinking more than two alcoholic drinks per day, estrogen deficiency (from removal of the ovaries or anti-breast cancer drugs), and vitamin D deficiency. Long periods of inactivity after your surgery or steroid drugs sometimes used with chemotherapy can also increase bone loss.

If you are on an AI, then you should follow a lifestyle that can help improve the strength of your bones. Lifestyle interventions include calcium and vitamin D supplements and weight-bearing exercises such as brisk walking for about 30 minutes four times a week. Sports like cycling or swimming, where your body weight is supported, are not weight-bearing and do not help with bone strength. Resistance exercise such as lifting light weights above your shoulders until your muscles are tired can also help. Flexibility-type exercises, such as yoga or tai chi, simple neck or shoulder rolls, and quadriceps or hamstring stretches are also thought to help prevent osteoporosis. To help prevent osteoporosis, eat calcium-rich foods such as cheese, milk, yogurt, nuts, tinned sardines and salmon, and dark green vegetables, as well as good sources of vitamin D such as salmon, mackerel, or fortified foods. Stop cigarette smoking and reduce or avoid sugar drinks and alcohol.

Drs. Chien and Goss, from the Massachusetts General Hospital, have advised the following (Chien 2006):

- A total calcium intake of 1,200–1,500 mg per day
- Vitamin D supplementation at 800 units per day
- Weight-bearing exercises
- Reduced alcohol consumption (no more than two drinks per day)
- Smoking cessation.

Some calcium and vitamin D combinations contain 600 mg of calcium and 500 mg of vitamin D and may not be enough, particularly if your vitamin D level is low; you may need to take two capsules a day. Supplements that only contain 200 units per day are not enough. Speak to your family doctor about this. If your vitamin D levels are very low, then your doctor may prescribe three to five tablets of 1,000 U per day (e.g. Ostelin) for six to 12 weeks to get the levels back to normal, and then a maintenance dose of 1,000 U per day would be required. Sources of calcium and vitamin D from the National Institutes of Health Office of Dietary management are shown in Tables 14 and 15 below and outlined at:

www.ods.od.nih.gov/Health_Information/Information_About_Individual_ Dietary_Supplements.aspx (US Department of Agriculture 2003, Pennington 1998 and 2004, Heaney 2000, Nutritional Coordination Center 2003).

Measurement equivalents and a useful conversion calculator can be found at the Exploratorium® website:

www.exploratorium.edu/cooking/convert/measurements.html

Tables 14 and 15 show that it is hard to get all your calcium and vitamin D from your diet. Very few foods in nature contain vitamin D, and you would also need two to three servings of milk, yoghurt, or cheese to reach your daily calcium allowance. Calcium and vitamin D supplements are therefore usually required, and of course a small amount of daily exposure to sunlight.

Food	Calcium (mg)	% Daily value
Yogurt, plain, low fat, 8 oz. (225 g)	415	42
Yogurt, fruit, low fat, 8 oz. (225 g)	245–384	25–38
Sardines, canned in oil, with bones, 3 oz. (85 g)	324	32
Cheddar cheese shredded, 1.5 oz. (43 g)	306	31
Milk, non-fat, 1 cup, 8 fl oz. (250 mL)	302	30
Milk, reduced fat (2% milk fat), no solids, 1 cup, 8 fl oz. (250 mL)	297	30
Milk, whole (3.25% milk fat), 1 cup, 8 fl oz. (250 mL)	291	29
Milk, buttermilk, 1 cup, 8 fl oz. (250 mL)	285	29
Milk, lactose reduced, 1 cup, 8 fl oz. (250 mL)	285–302	29–30
Mozzarella, part skim 1.5 oz. (43 g)	275	28
Orange juice, calcium fortified, 6 fl oz. (175 mL)	200–260	20–26
Salmon, pink, canned, solids with bone, 3 oz. (85 g)	181	18
Pudding, chocolate, instant, made w/ 2% milk, ½ cup, 4oz. (115 g)	153	15
Cottage cheese, 1% milk fat, 1 cup, 8 oz. (227 g)	138	14
Spinach, cooked, ½ cup, 4oz. (113 g)	120	12
Instant breakfast drink, powder prepared with water, 1 cup, 8 fl oz. (250 mL)	105–250	10–25
Frozen yogurt, vanilla, soft serve, ½ cup, 4oz. (113 g)	103	10
Ready to eat cereal, calcium fortified, 1 cup, 8oz. (227 g)	100–1,000	10–100
Turnip greens, boiled, ½ cup, 4oz. (113 g)	99	10
Kale (form of cabbage), cooked, 1 cup, 8oz. (227 g)	94	9
Ice cream, vanilla, ½ cup, 4oz. (113 g)	85	8.5
Soy beverage, calcium fortified, 1 cup, 8 fl oz. (250 mL)	80–500	8–50
Chinese cabbage, raw, 1 cup, 8oz. (227 g)	74	7
Tortilla, corn, ready to bake/fry, 1 medium	42	4
Tortilla, flour, ready to bake/fry, one 6" diameter	37	4
Sour cream, reduced fat, cultured, 2 tbsp, 1oz. (28 g)	32	3
Bread, white, 1 oz. (28 g)	31	3
Broccoli, raw, ½ cup, 4 oz. (113 g)	21	2
Bread, whole wheat, 1 slice	20	2
Cheese, cream, regular, 1 tbsp, 0.5 oz. (14 g)	12	1

Table 14: Selected food sources of calcium

Food	International Units per serving	% Daily value
Salmon, cooked, 3.5 oz. (105 g)	360	90
Mackerel, cooked, 3.5 oz. (105 g)	345	90
Tuna fish, canned in oil, 3 oz. (85 g)	200	50
Sardines, canned in oil, drained, 1.75 oz. (53 g)	250	70
Milk, non-fat, reduced fat, and whole, vitamin D-fortified, 1 cup, 8 fl oz. (250 mL)	98	25
Margarine, fortified, 1 tbsp, ½ oz. (14 g)	60	15
Ready-to-eat cereal, fortified with 10% of the DV for vitamin D, 1 cup, 8oz. (227 g)	40	10
Egg, 1 whole (vitamin D is found in yolk)	20	6
Liver, beef, cooked, 3.5 oz. (105 g)	15	4
Cheese, Swiss, 1 oz. (28 g)	12	4

Table 15: Selected food sources of vitamin D

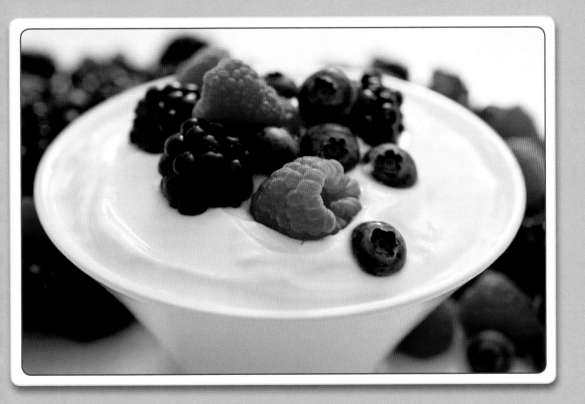

"Turning off" or removing the ovaries

"Turning off" or removing the ovaries lowers the level of estrogen in the blood if you have not gone through menopause. This is another way of "starving" estrogen receptor-positive cancer cells of estrogen to stop them from growing. Sometimes an AI is also added to bring about a "total estrogen blockade".

This treatment is not necessary if you have already gone through menopause because the ovaries naturally stop making estrogen after menopause. We sometimes recommend removal of the ovaries if you may be suspected of having or have a breast cancer gene that increases your risk of ovarian cancer.

Stopping the ovaries from working is never an easy decision, particularly if you're already on tamoxifen, since the additional benefit may not be worth all the menopausal side effects.

Turning off the ovaries with a medication: goserelin (Zoladex)

The ovaries can be shut down temporarily with medication. This is usually done with a course of monthly injections of goserelin (Zoladex). This gradually causes the levels of estrogen to fall, which leads to temporary menopause.

Zoladex works by reducing the levels of LH (luteinizing hormone) produced by the pituitary gland by interacting with a hormone in the hypothalamus (see Figure 82a). It is given by injection, usually every four weeks, just under the skin of the abdomen, by your doctor or nurse. Sometimes the injection is slightly uncomfortable and you may notice an area of redness or darker color in the surrounding skin afterwards.

Menstrual periods stop and other symptoms of menopause may develop (see below). These symptoms can be reversed. If the injections are stopped, estrogen levels and menstrual periods return to normal.

Some women who are considering having their ovaries removed will have these injections for a few months to "test out" the menopausal symptoms. They still have the choice of reversing the effect if the side effects are too intense. The use of goserelin is strictly controlled by governments in some countries—check with your doctor to see whether the government or your insurance company subsidizes these drugs or whether you'll have to pay for the injections yourself.

Zoladex is not a contraceptive. The risk of pregnancy is particularly high during initial treatment, so barrier methods of contraception such as condoms, IUDs, or diaphragms should be used during Zoladex treatment.

Surgical removal of the ovaries

The operation to remove the ovaries is called an **oophorectomy,** and is a permanent way to reduce estrogen levels. It is a very effective treatment for stopping early breast cancer from returning or for slowing the progress of metastatic cancer. It can also reduce the risk of ovarian cancer. For a long time in the 60s and 70s, it was the only form of treatment.

Removal of the ovaries can be done with keyhole surgery (using a laparoscope) or with an open operation (making an incision along the bikini line). We tend to use a keyhole approach because it's faster and has far fewer side effects. Usually the fallopian tubes are also removed, but the uterus (womb) is left intact.

After oophorectomy, the symptoms of menopause may come on suddenly. This is different than turning off the ovaries with medication, which brings menopausal symptoms on gradually. Obviously, there is no need for contraception after this.

Side effects of ovarian suppression or removal

Common side effects include:

- Symptoms of menopause, such as hot flashes, mood swings, difficulty sleeping, and vaginal dryness. These symptoms usually come on gradually over weeks or months after goserelin, as the levels of estrogen drop, or within a week or so after ovarian removal.

- Joint pains

- Weight gain can occur—you may gain a few pounds

- Thinning of the bones

- Tiredness—some women have less energy with lower levels of estrogen

- Your periods will stop, but goserelin may not be 100 percent effective as a contraceptive. Removing the ovaries will of course provide permanent contraception.

Turning off the ovaries after chemotherapy and tamoxifen

A very difficult decision is what to do if you are younger than 40 or so, have had a course of chemotherapy, have been started on tamoxifen because your tumor was estrogen sensitive, and then have your periods come back. The first control point here is—don't panic! It's not all that bad. Nobody really knows whether patients having chemotherapy and tamoxifen are better off having their ovaries removed. Evidence so far shows that the benefit is either small, negligible, or indeed zero. Peter Ravdin, in his online calculator for doctors, doesn't give the use of ovarian treatments any extra survival benefit over and above tamoxifen. Certainly if the chance of your cancer coming back is low anyway, then the extra theoretical benefit is likely to be negligible. The extra side effects from adding removal of the ovaries to chemotherapy and tamoxifen is probably not worth it in terms of your quality of life.

If you have lots of lymph glands involved with cancer and the chance of cancer coming back is higher, then maybe the pain is worth the potential gain. At this stage, the 15-year results from the Oxford meta-analysis or overview on this subject shows no added benefit from stopping the ovaries from working.

Once again, go with your gut feeling, because if you are young and have already had a lot of chemotherapy and tamoxifen and really don't want to go through an irreversible menopause, you may wish to consider waiting for your periods to stop naturally or having a reversible injection such as goserelin to stop your periods, thus giving yourself a test run before having your ovaries removed. There are several ongoing trials that may answer this question for sure in the future.

CONTROL POINT #16 – DO I NEED HORMONAL TREATMENT?

WARNING It's a good idea to stop your hormonal treatments about one week before flying long distances or if you are immobilized for a time after any future surgery, as they may increase your chance of blood clots in your legs.

TIP If you have an estrogen receptor-positive tumor, hormonal treatments such as tamoxifen or an aromatase inhibitor are usually given after your other treatments (radiation therapy or chemotherapy) have finished.

REMEMBER Hormonal treatments for breast cancer are not contraceptives. They have been used for many years and have been found to be very effective in reducing the risk of cancer coming back after surgery.

Mays Story

In 1999 on New Year's Eve in San Francisco May being 89 years of age was dancing in the street with her granddaughter when she first felt a lump in the upper part of her right breast in her arm pit.

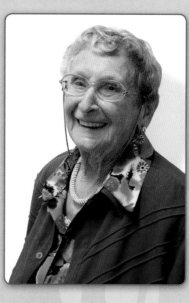

May was a professional dancer all her life and decided she was far too busy to see a doctor. At that time she was teaching the "Rookwood Rockers", an entertainment group for older people in nursing homes.

Every week May and her troupe would go to different nursing home and tap dance and entertain the old folk.

In 2003 when May was 92 she finally had time to see us in the clinic. She saw our surgeon first and then she saw me on the same day. Our surgeon recommended a mastectomy as this was a quicker and easier treatment at the age of 92.

I sat with May and asked her what she did in her spare time and May said she was a dancer, particularly tap dancing. I then said "May, your breasts are very important to you then" and she said "you bet they are!"

I quietly negotiated with our surgeon that a tablet was probably the best thing to do and I started May on Femara, an aromatase inhibitor.

May is now 99 years old and going well and her cancer has shrunk from 5cm in March 2003 to just under 2cms in March 2010. May is taking is easy these days but still lives an active life, and pleased that she didn't have her breast removed.

In May's view it was "try the tablets first before you have it off, when you're my age".

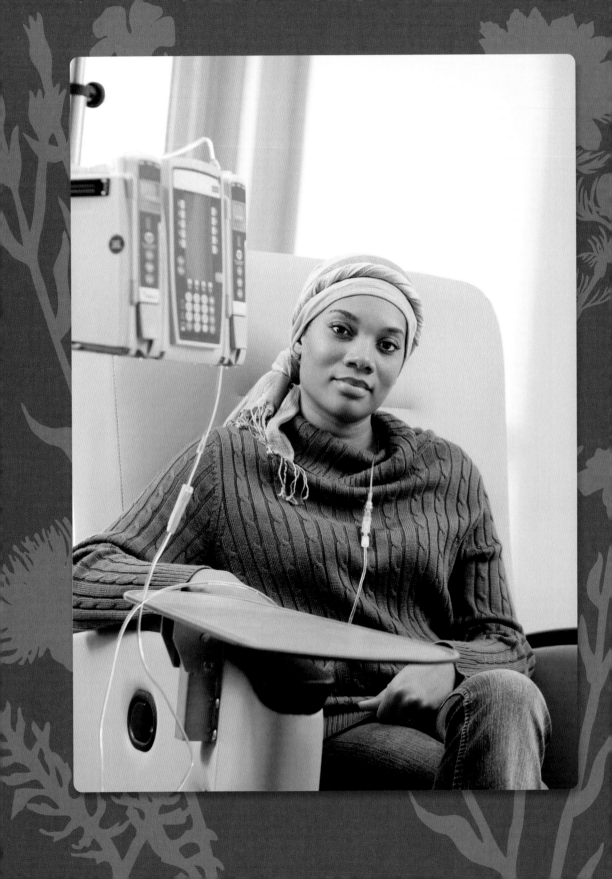

Control Point 17

Do I Need Chemotherapy?

Control Point #17

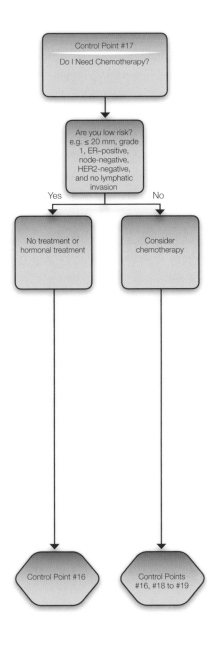

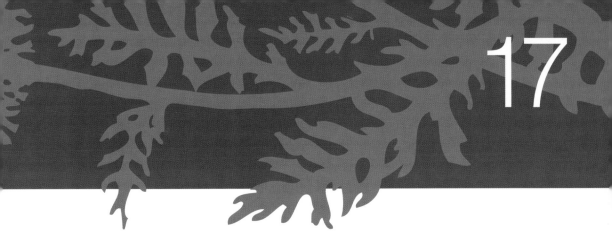

Do I Need Chemotherapy?

What is "adjuvant" chemotherapy and how does it work?

The trouble with cancer cells is that you need a special microscope to see them, and our scans cannot detect whether cells have left the breast or the gland area and traveled to another area, unless those cells have formed clumps at least the size of a small cherry. As mentioned in the previous chapter, it makes good sense to treat cells that may have already spread beyond the breast and glands sooner rather than later.

To reiterate my garden example, if a particular weed in the first garden patch under the rose bush looks like it may be delicate enough to blow easily in the wind to other parts of the garden, then it's best to use weed killer now and prevent the seed from sprouting (Figure 80). In many situations, it's best if we use chemotherapy, particularly if your breast cancer cell is not sensitive to estrogen.

Chemotherapy is an additional (or "adjuvant") medication that treats undetectable cancer cells that may be in another part of the body. Chemotherapy is also called "chemo," and another medical word for it is "cytotoxic drugs." They are also called "anti-cancer drugs". Sometimes we use "neo-adjuvant" chemotherapy, which is where we give chemotherapy before surgery or radiation therapy for larger, more advanced cancers.

Chemotherapy works against dividing cells. Most of the cells in our body go through what is called the cell cycle, in which a cell divides into two identical cells with their own set of DNA. Chemotherapy drugs interfere with various parts of this cycle so that the cells can't divide or repair themselves if damaged. Normal, non-cancerous cells have a better ability to repair themselves.

Therefore, chemotherapy works against all cells that divide—both normal and cancer cells. Cells that divide include your hair (and that's why you need a haircut every so often), your nails, your bone marrow, and the lining of your mouth and bowel. Skin also divides, and all of these parts of your body can be affected by chemotherapy.

There are more than 20 possible combinations of chemotherapy, and different drugs have different side effects. It's impossible to summarize all the different types in this book, but your doctor will explain which "recipe" he or she he use in your situation and why.

Very early studies done in the 70s, particularly from Milan in Italy, showed that giving even one course of chemotherapy can reduce the chance of your breast cancer coming back. Over the next 30 years, there have been various "generations" of chemotherapy. Just like cars have improved over the last 30 years, so has chemotherapy and the associated drugs that prevent or lessen side effects such as nausea and vomiting.

Unfortunately, most chemotherapy agents still cause your hair to be lost for a little while. This is the hardest part of the treatment, particularly because it's a very visible, obvious statement that you have had cancer.

By how much does chemotherapy improve my chances?

This is a very difficult question to answer and to a large extent it depends on how good or not your prognosis is to start with. The Adjuvant! Online calculator I showed you earlier can help your doctor work it out for your own set of circumstances (Figure 72). The important points are as follows:

- Chemotherapy does help—sometimes a little and sometimes a lot

- Chemotherapy reduces the risk of dying from breast cancer from as little as 1 to 2 percent to as much as 20 to 30 percent. However, watch this type of statistic as explained in Table 11 above

- The older you are, the less likely it is that chemotherapy will be helpful

- The older you are, the more likely it is that hormonal treatment will be useful

- If your tumor is hormone sensitive, hormonal treatment is also very important and gives additional benefit, over and above the benefit of chemotherapy

- Sometimes when a tumor is hormone sensitive, hormonal treatment alone may be better than chemotherapy alone, or nearly as good as hormonal treatment and chemotherapy. Ask your doctor to list the benefits from hormonal treatment alone or hormonal treatment with chemotherapy.

- Always look at your options, balance the good and bad effects of chemotherapy, and take your time to make your decision

- Chemotherapy does not guarantee that your cancer will be cured, but it can improve your odds.

But remember, it's all about balancing your odds with the risks and benefits of chemotherapy. It's a bit like giving a racehorse a steroid to give it a greater chance of winning—it might have won the race in any case.

Another analogy we sometimes use is airbags in cars. Giving extra treatments is like having some driver's-side airbags. Sometimes, more intensive chemo is like putting airbags in the side doors and car roof. Sometimes this is not worth the extra cost, and sometimes it is. Firstly, find out what your chances of having an "accident" are, and then the extra chance of surviving it if you have airbags.

Don't feel too guilty if you just "buy" half the available airbags and maybe reduce your chances by 1 or 2 percent. However, many of our patients do want absolutely everything done, and this is okay as well. In this case, the short-term pain may be worth the long-term gain.

When is chemotherapy given in relation to all my other treatments?

If chemotherapy is given, generally there are three to four possible approaches. The actual approach may depend on the policies, routines, and experience of your medical oncologist and your radiation oncologist (Figure 86). Usually, some blood tests and a baseline heart scan may be done, as very rarely, some chemotherapy agents called "anthracyclines" which include doxorubicin (Adriamycin) or epirubicin (Ellence) can cause heart damage. Your oncologist will want to make sure your heart is functioning normally before he or she recommends these drugs. Chemotherapy normally would start at week three or four following surgery.

TREATMENT STRATEGY

WEEK	A	B	C	D	E	F	G	H	I	J
1	CS	CS	CS	CS	CS	CS	CS	M	M	M
2										
3	PO	PO	PO	PO	PO	PO	PO	PO	PO	PO
4	SIM								SIM	
5		CT	CT	CT	CT	CT	CT	HT		CT
6	RT								RT	
7	RT								RT	
8	RT	CT	CT	CT	CT	CT	CT		RT	CT
9	RT								RT	
10	RT								RT	
11	RT	CT	CT	CT	CT	CT	CT		HT	CT
12	HT									
13		SIM		SIM	SIM	SIM				
14		CT	CT	CT	CT	CT	CT			CT
15										HT
16										
17		RT	CT	RT	RT	RT	CT			
18		RT		RT	RT	RT				
19		RT	SIM	RT	RT	RT				
20		RT	CT	RT	RT	RT	CT			
21		RT		RT	RT	RT				
22		RT		RT	RT	RT				
23		HT	RT				CT			
24			RT							
25			RT	CT	CT	CT				
26			RT	CT	CT		CT			
27			RT	CT	CT					
28			RT	CT	CT	CT				
29			HT	CT	CT		RT			
30				CT	CT		RT			
31				CT	CT	CT	RT			
32				CT	CT		RT			
33				HT	CT		RT			
34					CT	CT	RT			
35					CT	HT	HT			
36					CT					
37					HT					

CS	CONSERVATIVE SURGERY
CT	CHEMOTHERAPY CYCLE GIVEN
RT	RADIATION GIVEN
PO	FIRST POST-OPERATIVE VISIT
HT	HORMONAL TREATMENT COMMENCES

Figure 86: Timing of surgery, radiation therapy, chemotherapy and hormonal treatment.

TREATMENT STRATEGY

WEEK	K	L	M	N	O	P	Q	R	S	T
1	M	M	M	M	M	M	M	M+IR	M+IR	M+IR
2										
3	PO	PO	PO	PO	PO	PO	PO	PO	PO	PO
4									E	E
5	CT	CT	CT	CT	CT	CT	CT	CT	CT	HT
6									E	E
7							CT			
8	CT	CT	CT	CT	CT	CT		CT	CT	
9							CT		E	E
10										
11	CT	CT	CT	CT	CT	CT	CT	CT	CT	
12									E	E
13			SIM	SIM	SIM	SIM	CT	SIM	SIM	
14	CT	CT	CT	CT	CT	CT		CT	CT	
15							CT		E	E
16									HT	
17	CT	CT	RT	RT	RT	RT	CT	RT		
18			RT	RT	RT	RT		RT		
19		SIM	RT	RT	RT	RT	CT	RT		
20	CT	CT	RT	RT	RT	RT	HT	RT		
21	HT		RT	RT	RT	RT		RT		
22						HT		HT		
23		RT								
24		RT	CT	CT	CT					
25		RT	CT	CT						
26		RT	CT	CT						
27		RT	CT	CT	CT					
28		HT	CT	CT					PI	PI
29			CT	CT						
30			CT	CT	CT					
31			CT	CT						
32			HT	CT						
33				CT	CT					
34				CT	HT					
35				CT						
36				HT				PI		
37										

M	MASTECTOMY
M+IR	MASTECTOMY AND IMMEDIATE (IMPLANT) RECONSTRUCTION
E	EXPANSION OF IMPLANT
PI	PERMANENT IMPLANT
SIM	RADIATION SIMULATION AND PLANNING

Chemotherapy after breast conservation

If you are having a lumpectomy and radiation therapy, there are three basic approaches to integrate chemotherapy with your other treatments:

- Give all the chemotherapy first (e.g. four to eight cycles of chemotherapy once every three weeks). Three weeks after the last course of chemo, your radiation therapy will commence (Figure 86, treatment strategies B, C and G).

- If you have a lot of lymph glands involved in your armpit, chemotherapy can be given before radiation therapy for four to six cycles, followed by the radiation therapy, followed by four to 12 additional cycles of chemotherapy (the "sandwich approach") (Figure 86, treatment strategies D, E and F).

- In the early years, we did give chemotherapy at the same time as radiation therapy. Although this is still possible, the treatment is harder, both with trying to get to multiple appointments and with side effects, such as increased skin reaction and fatigue. Further, some of my previous research has shown that there is a higher incidence of inflammation of the lung if chemotherapy is given at the same time as radiation therapy.

In Figure 86, radiation is given for six weeks if breast conservation is done (five weeks to the breast and then a one-week boost to the scar) and for five weeks after a mastectomy.

Chemotherapy after a mastectomy with no radiation therapy

If chemotherapy is given after a mastectomy, most oncologists wait three to four weeks to allow you to recover from your surgery and get your arm moving again. If no chemotherapy is given, you may start hormonal treatment about one to three weeks after your mastectomy (Figure 86, treatment strategy H). Generally, chemotherapy is given every three weeks for approximately four to six courses, as shown in Figure 86, treatment strategies J and K.

With the advent of drugs to support the bone marrow (particularly the white cells, which fight infection), "dose-dense" treatments every two weeks rather than the more common frequency of every three weeks are also being tested and increasingly being used in clinical practice (Figure 86, treatment strategy Q) for a patient having a mastectomy.

Chemotherapy after a mastectomy with radiation therapy

Generally, there are two approaches. Either all the chemotherapy can be given first and then be followed by radiation therapy (treatment strategies L and P) or we can use the "sandwich approach," wherein we give three to six cycles of chemotherapy first, followed by five weeks of radiation therapy, followed by four to 12 additional cycles of chemotherapy (treatment strategies M, N and 0).

Chemotherapy after a mastectomy, if a reconstruction is done and radiation is given

The timing of treatments if reconstruction is required can be complicated and will vary from center to center. The approach that I follow is outlined in Figure 86 above (treatment strategies R, S and T). In our practice, we inflate the implant between courses of chemotherapy and have it totally inflated before radiation is planned.

Some centers deflate the implant before radiation is given. This makes the radiotherapy planning process less complicated and allows better coverage of areas such as the lymph glands behind the breastbone. The implant can then be re-inflated about six to eight weeks later when the radiotherapy skin changes have settled down.

Types of chemotherapy

There are probably over 30 different adjuvant chemotherapy recipes or "regimens "in use. Deciding which treatment to pursue is quite complex and often involves some uncertainty. Always discuss this with your treatment team and of course your family.

I like Peter Ravdin's summary in his Adjuvant! Online program. Peter has grouped adjuvant chemotherapy into "generations," defined by efficacy and toxicity. He has also documented the "relative risk" of dying by each generation to work out what the "absolute" survival benefit is for your type of tumor. The absolute risk is the easiest to understand, and this is what can be printed for you by your doctors (see Control Point #15 - What Do the Statistics Really Mean?).

In general, the third generation drugs are slightly better but have more side effects than the first generation drugs, and have usually been discovered more recently.

It's about getting the balance right. In general, if your prognosis is relatively good, there's not a lot to gain from having third generation chemotherapy. You may only need hormonal treatment or no treatment for the whole body at all. If your disease is more serious, then stronger and longer treatment is probably better.

Most specialists and doctors are genuinely trying to help you, so don't be afraid to ask them questions about the minimum number of courses you need and whether or not the number of courses can be cut back. Usually, if your prognosis is considered better, shorter courses are given, and sometimes the number of courses may be cut back if you get unexpected side effects.

Defining the "generations" of chemotherapy

Table 16 gives a summary of the different types of chemotherapy treatments classified by generations.

First generation:

- Generally modest toxicity
- Moderate reduction in the risk of dying
- Common drugs used include:
  - C = cyclophosphamide (Cytoxan): this can be given intravenously (IV) or orally

- M = methotrexate (Mexate): IV
- F = 5-FU or 5-fluorouracil (Adrucil): IV
- E = epirubicin (Ellence): IV
- A = doxorubicin (Adriamycin): IV

A number in parentheses such as "(50)" generally means the dose given, adjusted for your weight and height (referred to as a dose of 50 milligrams [mg] per meter squared). The notation "FE(50)C x 6" above means the three drugs (5-FU, epirubicin (at 50 mg/m2), and cyclophosphamide) given for six courses or cycles.

Second generation:

- More effective than first-generation drugs
- Generally longer in duration and with more side effects than first generation regimens
- Greater reduction in the risk of dying
- Common drugs used include:

- F = 5-FU or 5-fluorouracil: IV
- E = epirubicin (Ellence): IV
- C = cyclophosphamide (Cytoxan): IV
- T = paclitaxel (Taxol): IV
- A = doxorubicin (Adriamycin): IV

Third generation:

- More effective that first- or second-generation drugs

- Usually have more risk of infection, but this is often prevented with antibiotics and using drugs that boost your white cells, such as Neulasta

- Common drugs used include:

  - T = paclitaxel (Taxol): IV

- D = docetaxel (Taxotere, often referred to as "T"): IV

- A = doxorubicin (Adriamycin): IV

- C = cyclophosphamide (Cytoxan): IV

- F = 5-FU or 5-fluorouracil (Adrucil): IV

- E = epirubicin (Ellence): IV

This way of organizing regimens by generations brings some order to our thinking about different chemotherapy treatments that have never been directly compared.

The choice of chemotherapy will to a large extent depend on your oncologist, who will use a combination of factors but particularly your cancer's estrogen receptor (ER) status and HER-2 status, to work out the best regimen or "recipe" for your own individual circumstances. You may be asked to be part of a clinical trial where you will be "randomized" (where choice of treatment is allocated between two or more different treatments) between standard therapy and a new treatment being tested. Don't be afraid to participate in a trial. It often means access to better treatment and more specialized care, sometimes at a lower or no cost, and it may help people in the future too.

In 2009, the National Comprehensive Cancer Network recommended the following regimens as "preferred" but noted that the selection, dosing, and administration of anti-cancer agents is complex. There is no real correct answer, to be honest, and they mentioned other regimens too, including FAC and FEC. Here are the "preferred" regimens:

Without Herceptin (trastuzumab)

- TAC (docetaxel/doxorubicin/cyclophosphamide) every 21 days for six cycles

- Dose-dense AC (doxorubicin/cyclophosphamide) followed by paclitaxel every 14 days for four cycles

- AC (doxorubicin/cyclophosphamide) every 21 days for four cycles, followed by weekly paclitaxel for 12 cycles

- TC (docetaxel and cyclophosphamide) every 21 days for four cycles

- AC (doxorubicin/cyclophosphamide) every 21 days for four cycles

Acronym and number of courses	Drugs Used	Generation
AC x 4	doxorubicin (A)/cyclophosphamide (C) every three weeks	1
CMF x 6	cyclophosphamide (C) (oral) (days 1-14)/methotrexate (M)/fluorouracil (F) days 1 and 8 every 4 weeks	1
EC x 4	epirubicin (E)/cyclophosphamide (C) every three weeks	1
FE(50)C x 6	fluorouracil (F)/epirubicin (E) (50 mg per m^2)/cyclophosphamide (C) every three weeks	1
AC x 4 then T x 4	doxorubicin(A)/cyclophosphamide (C) followed by sequential paclitaxel (T) x 4, every three weeks (or weekly T x 8–12)	2
E(100) x 4 then CMF x 4	epirubicin (E) (100 mg per m^2) three weekly followed by cyclophosphamide(C)/methotrexate (M)/fluorouracil (F) (as above, but four instead of six courses)	2
FAC x 6	fluorouracil (F)/doxorubicin (A)/cyclophosphamide (C) every three weeks	2
FE(100)C x 6	fluorouracil (F)/epirubicin (E) (100 mg per m^2)/cyclophosphamide (C); also known as "FEC-100," every three weeks	2
DC x 4	docetaxel(D) (Taxotere) and cyclophosphamide (C) every three weeks	2
FE(100)C x 3 then D x 3	cyclophosphamide (C)/epirubicin (E) (100 mg per m^2)/fluorouracil (F)x 3 then docetaxel (D)(100 mg/m^2) x 3, every three weeks	3
A then T then C	doxorubicin followed by paclitaxel (T) followed by cyclophosphamide (C), every two weeks with filgrastim support	3
AC x 4 then T x 4	doxorubicin (A)/cyclophosphamide (C) followed by sequential paclitaxel (T) x 4, every two weeks	3
FE(90–100) C x 4 then T x 8–12 (weekly)	fluorouracil (F)/epirubicin (E) (90–100 mg per m^2)/cyclophosphamide (C) every three weeks followed by docetaxel weekly for 8–12 courses	3
DAC (usually known as "TAC") x 6	docetaxel (D)/doxorubicin (A)/cyclophosphamide (C) every three weeks	3

Table 16: Examples of different "generations" of chemotherapy

With Herceptin (trastuzumab)

- AC (doxorubicin/ cyclophosphamide) every 21 days for four cycles, followed by weekly paclitaxel for 12 cycles or every paclitaxel every 21 days for four cycles with trastuzumab for one year

- Dose-dense AC (doxorubicin/ cyclophosphamide), followed by paclitaxel every 14 days for four cycles with trastuzumab for one year

- TCH (docetaxel, carboplatin) every 21 days for four cycles, followed by trastuzumab for one year

Understanding the benefit of chemotherapy

There are too many combinations to work out your own situation. Ask your doctor to do this on his or her computer.

The bottom line is that the more advanced your disease is (the larger it is or the more lymph glands involved), the greater the benefit of a higher generation of treatment. Below is an example using the following scenario:

- Age = 50

- Tumor size = 20 mm

- Nodal status = negative

- Grade = 2

- Estrogen receptor status = positive

- The baseline prognosis at ten years

96.2 percent

without any treatment = 92.0 percent

- Adding five years of tamoxifen or another hormonal treatment adds 2.4 percent = 94.4 percent

- Adding **CMF** (generation 1 chemo) and tamoxifen adds a total of 3.3 percent = 95.3 percent

- Adding generation 2 chemo and tamoxifen gives a total benefit of

- Adding generation 3 chemo and tamoxifen gives a total benefit of 96.9 percent

As you can see, there's not much difference between the treatments, and I would probably err on the side of recommending just some tamoxifen, which gives a ten-year survival rate of 94.4 percent—1.8 percent less than second generation chemo or if you really want to have some extra benefit from chemotherapy maybe, first generation chemotherapy is probably adequate.

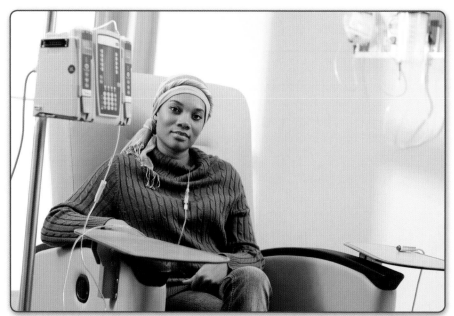

Figure 87: Most chemotherapy agents are given through a vein using an intravenous line. Take someone along to support you.

If your disease is more advanced, then you're probably better off with second or third generation chemotherapy agents. For the same characteristics above but with more than nine nodes involved:

- The baseline survival is about 50-50 at ten years (45 percent)

- Tamoxifen alone only gives an extra 13.1 percent (not enough)

- Generation 1 chemo and tamoxifen adds 18.3 percent (getting better)

- Generation 3 chemo is looking better; it adds 29.1 percent (much better)

- Maximum ten year survival with third generation chemotherapy and tamoxifen in this scenario is 74 percent.

So, if the disease is more extensive, then the pain is probably worth the gain. If it's early (maybe fewer than four lymph glands involved), third generation chemo is not much better than first or second generation chemo with tamoxifen.

Your own doctor will have the recipes that he or she is most comfortable with, but it's important that you aren't over-treated or under-treated.

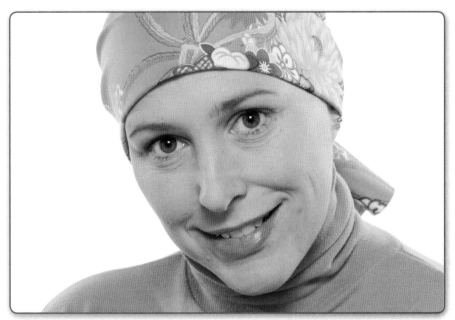

Figure 88: Chemotherapy turbans, scarves, caps, or head wraps are an alternative to wigs.

How is chemotherapy given?

Most chemotherapy agents are given through a vein using an intravenous line. This is often called an IV in medical jargon. Usually, you will need to see the doctor, who will check your blood tests. This visit usually takes place a week or so before your next chemotherapy course is due. Having chemotherapy on a Friday gives you a couple of days when family is home on the weekend to help you recover, and you may be well enough to get back to work on Monday or Tuesday. Unless you are in the hospital, you don't need to wear a gown and can just wear your normal clothes. Wearing a loose fitting top will allow the nurses to access your arm for the chemotherapy injection. The nurses will wear protective gowns and gloves.

When you come for chemotherapy, it's best to ask a friend or a family member to come with you, not only for moral support but also to help you drive home. Sometimes the anti-nausea medication can affect your driving. Check with your oncologist on this one. If you find that the anti-nausea drugs they use didn't make you drowsy and you coped well after your first treatment, then you may be all right to drive home on your own.

It's also a good idea to bring a book, an MP3 player or iPod, or even a portable DVD player to help make the time go faster and help you relax. Bring a water bottle to stay hydrated.

If the blood test is done on the same day as the chemotherapy, this will be checked, and then a decision will be made about whether the treatment will go ahead. If your blood count is a little low (remember that your bone marrow is also a dividing cell), then the oncologist may drop the dose a little or, more often than not, postpone the treatment for a week or two.

If your test results are acceptable, then an intravenous line will be inserted into one of your veins. With experienced chemotherapy nurses, this only takes a few seconds and there will only be a little pinprick.

Sometimes, veins do get damaged from more and more needles, making them difficult to find. Some drugs can be very damaging to the skin if the vein is damaged and the chemotherapy agent leaks around the vein under your skin (e.g. doxorubicin or epirubicin). This is called **extravasation**, and there are procedures to reduce the risk of complications if this occurs. Some drugs just cause irritation and may cause some skin pigmentation or hardening of the veins around the injection site.

Sometimes, your veins may be deep and difficult to find, and in some situations, your doctor may recommend some sort of **port** where a permanent line is inserted into one of your large veins (Figure 87). This makes it a lot easier for both drawing blood and giving you chemotherapy.

Seriously consider a port if you are having more than six courses of chemotherapy. Ports can be removed after chemotherapy is completed, and the rates of complications from ports, which include bruising and rarely infection, are very, very low.

Side effects of chemotherapy

There are always extremes with chemotherapy. A few patients get very severe side effects and really don't want to come back. This is very rare these days with the type of medicines we have to stop nausea and vomiting. Drinking lots of fluids after your chemotherapy for two to three days has been found to be helpful.

Other patients have absolutely no side effects. The majority of patients do get some side effects, and sometimes these can snowball and become a bit worse with the more cycles of chemotherapy that you have. You will hear horror stories from other people and their reports of side effects from 20 or 30 years ago. Remember that our drugs have changed dramatically, and there are often solutions to any side effects that you may have.

Always talk to your chemotherapy nursing team and your doctors to ensure that you have a tolerable experience. It is important not to suffer in silence, as there are often ways of relieving many of the side effects of chemotherapy.

Hair Loss

This is the most distressing of all side effects, in my experience. Your hair is a statement of you and your personality, and losing it is often a public statement that you have cancer. Some of what we call our first generation drugs (e.g. CMF), particularly when given intravenously, only caused hair thinning over the course of your treatment.

Regimens such AC cause complete loss of scalp hair, over a few days, about two to three weeks after your first course of treatment starts. AC can sometimes cause loss of eyebrows, eyelashes and pubic hair.

The stronger, more recent second and third generation drugs (e.g. TAC) almost inevitably make you lose all your hair, including your eyelashes and pubic hair in the same period of time as AC.

The medical term for hair loss is **alopecia**. Remember that your hair always grows back, often thicker and curlier but, depending on your age, also grayer. Keep in mind the following:

- Your hair always grows back

- Consider buying a wig before your hair falls out so that your wig specialist can look at what your hair normally looks like

- Your hair begins to fall out by the second or third week of chemotherapy. Sometimes it comes out in clumps, and with some drugs, like the taxanes, it may come out all at once.

- You may experience scalp pain, tenderness, or itching for a few days before your hair starts to fall out

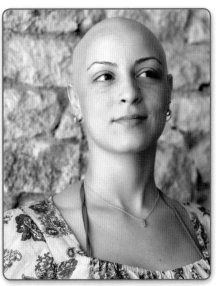

Figure 89: A few women prefer no headwear after chemotherapy.

- Many women find clumps of hair in their shower or on their pillow, and this can be distressing. Consider cutting your hair short to avoid the stress of large locks of hair falling out.

- Look at the *Look Good Feel Better* Program, which gives advice about how to manage your skin and cosmetics during your treatment. See www.lookgoodfeelbetter.org.

- Consider a wig, a bandana, scarf, head wrap or a beanie (Figure 88)

- A few brave and confident women prefer to wear no headwear (see Figure 89 and Bec's Story)

- If you lose your eyebrows, you can thicken them with pencil

- The hair starts to grow back about three weeks after your chemotherapy ends

- Your hair will grow at about 0.2 to 0.4 inches (or 5 to 10 mm) per month and can come back curly ("chemo curls"), a different color, or gray

- After some chemotherapy agents (e.g. weekly Taxol), the hair may start growing back immediately.

I normally recommend that my patients dye their hair, if it comes back gray, as soon as possible after it grows back. There seems to be a lot of mixed advice about this, and some people caution against it, but I find that it gives women a very fast psychological boost. See your hairdresser about using some sort of color that isn't too harsh on the hair and scalp.

You also need to take care of your scalp. Very occasionally, you may be allergic to the backing material of your wig, and a moisturizer or some steroid cream may be needed. Keep your scalp moisturized at all times, because it can get dry. You will also feel the cold through your scalp and you may need to wear a turban or cap if you're not wearing your wig. It's also a good idea to wash and massage your scalp with some gentle shampoo to clear away any dirt and scaly skin so that your new hair will be ready to grow back once your treatment is over.

In Australia, to find out where to get wigs and turbans, call the Cancer Council Helpline on 13 11 20. In the US, look at the Breast Cancer Network of Strength (formerly known as Y-Me) national support organization, www.networkofstrength.org, which can send wigs to women with hair loss for a nominal fee. In addition, the Breast Cancer Network Australia has developed an excellent fact sheet on hair loss, found at:

www.bcna.org.au/content/view/669/1280/

A great site in the UK about wigs and hair care is found here:

www.cancerhelp.org.uk/help/default.asp?page=13501

Skin and nail changes

Minor skin problems can occur while you are having chemotherapy. Possible changes include itching, redness, dryness, peeling, and acne. For itching and dryness, take quick, cooler showers or sponge yourself rather than taking long, hot baths. Apply cream and lotion and avoid perfume that contains alcohol. If you develop acne, try to keep your face dry and clean and use over-the-counter medicated creams or soaps.

Sometimes chemotherapy may cause darkening of the skin along the vein into which it was given, and makeup can be used to cover the area until it fades over the next few months. Chemotherapy can make you extra sensitive to the sun, so use a mild (baby type) sunscreen lotion when out in the sun, and wear protective hats and clothing.

Some people who have had radiation therapy before may develop "radiation recall" during their chemotherapy: during or shortly after anticancer drugs are given, the skin over the area that was treated with radiation turns red again. Check with your doctor, who needs to check whether the symptoms are caused by an infection (in which case you may have a temperature). If you feel well and don't have a temperature, apply the creams you were using during your radiation therapy.

Your nails may become brittle and darken a little, develop ridges, and could crack. The delay in nail growth from the chemotherapy may create vertical lines or bands. These changes usually grow out after the treatment has finished. Nail hardeners may help with nail changes, and wearing gloves when washing dishes or gardening may also help.

Nausea and vomiting

Not everyone feels sick after chemotherapy. It generally happens a few hours after the chemotherapy, but it does vary according to the drug. The nausea can sometimes start the next day. It sometimes feels like morning sickness. There are various ways of trying to help with nausea, including:

- Avoid fried or other fatty foods

- Avoid a totally empty stomach when you go for chemotherapy. Some dry crackers or a very light non-fatty snack may help.

- Avoid eating your favorite foods when you're nauseated so you don't develop an aversion to them

- Try breathing through your mouth when you feel nauseated

- If the smell of food makes you nauseated, take a walk while food is being prepared

- Your doctor may prescribe some anti-nausea pills, such as ondansetron (Zofran), for 24 to 48 hours after treatment to prevent nausea and vomiting.

The National Cancer Institute has published guidelines on how to manage nausea and vomiting after chemotherapy.

www.cancer.gov/cancertopics/pdq/supportivecare/nausea/patient

There is a type of vomiting called anticipatory vomiting. This is the feeling of nausea and vomiting when you return to the chemotherapy ward, with its associated smells and visual reminders. I had one patient who had to see me in a different facility because even the color of the walls and the carpets reminded her of chemotherapy.

Drugs used to prevent nausea include:

- ondansetron (Zofran)

- dolasetron (Anzemet)

- granisetron (Kytril)

- prochlorperazine (Stemetil, Buccastem, Compazine)

- dimenhydrinate (Gravol, Dramamine)

- metoclopramide (Maxeran, Reglan, Maxolon, Primperan)

- haloperidol (Haldol)

- nabilone (Cesamet)

- aprepitant (Emend)

- dexamethasone (Decadron)

- lorazepam (Ativan)

Some of these drugs can cause side effects themselves. Zofran may cause some headaches and constipation, and Stemetil and Maxolon can cause some restlessness and tremor.

Some of these drugs can also be used as anal suppositories, which may make it easier if you have vomited or are nauseated. Just ask the nurse for some disposable gloves; these generally slip in quite easily. Some patients have found that flat ginger beer or ale can ease nausea as well.

Chemotherapy effect on the blood cells

The reason we give chemotherapy every three weeks is so that your bone marrow, which is like a little factory that produces blood cells, has a chance to catch up and regenerate all your normal cells.

The important cells in the blood are the white cells, which fight infection; the red cells, which bring oxygen to your cells; and the platelets, which help clotting and stop bruising.

The most common effect of chemotherapy is a reduction in the white cells. The maximum effect occurs two weeks after treatment, and it is at that time that you're most prone to infection. Low white cells is called **neutropenia**, low red cells is **anemia**, and low platelets is called **thrombocytopenia.**

Avoid people who have obvious infections (who are coughing or sneezing), but there is no need to avoid people in general or to avoid crowded areas. You can have the injectable form of flu vaccine but the US Department of Health & Human Services recommends that anyone with a weakened immune system avoid the nasal spray flu vaccine which contains weakened live flu viruses. If your doctor advises the flu vaccine during treatment have the injection on the day before your next course and check that your white cell count is normal. There are no problems with the injectable flu vaccine if you are just having radiotherapy or hormonal treatment.

If you are not feeling well, check your temperature with a thermometer and follow your doctor's advice if it is over 38° Celsius or 100.5 degrees Fahrenheit. If you get a fever, sweats, chills, a cough with yellow sputum, burning urine, a sore that won't heal, or diarrhea that won't settle down, **call your doctor immediately** so that antibiotics can be prescribed.

Sometimes, you may need to be admitted to the hospital for five to seven days while you receive intravenous antibiotics, if you get a severe infection when you don't have the white blood cells, called neutrophils, that fight infection. This is called "neutropenic sepsis" or "febrile neutropenia" and can be life threatening if not treated in a hospital as soon as possible.

Some doctors recommend a substance called a granulocyte colony stimulating factor (G-CSF), such as filgrastim (Neupogen) or pegfilgrastim (Neulasta), which may help to reduce the chance of your white cells dropping too low. These are administered by yourself or a nurse, via an injection under the skin (like insulin for diabetics), 24 hours after your chemotherapy. These drugs are very important if you're having a third generation chemotherapy protocol, but check with your doctor regarding insurance or government restrictions on filgrastim or pegfilgrastim.

Filgrastim can accelerate recovery of your white cells, leading to a reduction in duration of the time that your neutrophils remain low. The neutrophils are at their lowest point two weeks after your chemotherapy. If you get a high temperature at any time during your treatment course, but particularly two weeks after your dose of chemotherapy, see your doctor immediately and call your oncology center.

Anemia, a reduction in your blood's ability to carry oxygen to the cells in your body, may cause you to feel a bit dizzy, short of breath, and tired. It's not very common, but if it occurs, it's not usually helped by taking iron or vitamin B. The quickest way to fix this is with a blood transfusion. Although some doctors may give a hormone injection called erythropoietin (EPO) a try, concerns have been raised about its usefulness for patients with cancer due to speculation that these agents may cause blood clots and possibly even tumor growth (Bohlius 2006, Murray 2008).

Low platelet counts are a rare side effect. Drugs like aspirin can affect platelet function, so it's best to avoid aspirin during chemotherapy and just stick to drugs such as Tylenol/Panadol. Leukemia has been reported after chemotherapy, but the risk is very low and occurs in fewer than one in 200 to 300 patients who have chemotherapy. Overall, the benefit of chemotherapy outweighs this risk (Hudis 2002).

Diarrhea or constipation

Don't be alarmed by minor effects on your bowel. They usually settle down. If you develop severe diarrhea that persists for more than 24 hours, though, make sure that you go to the hospital for a check. Sometimes you can get dehydrated. Although this is rare, it's important that you have access to fluids if it occurs, and sometimes these need to be given intravenously. If it is severe, then a test of your stool may be necessary to work out if there's a bug that needs to be targeted with a specific antibiotic.

While you're having chemotherapy, avoid foods that can increase bowel function, such as cabbage, beans, high fiber foods, and also spicy foods. Reducing your consumption of milk may also help reduce diarrhea, particularly if you are slightly milk (or lactose) intolerant.

Some chemotherapy drugs can cause constipation, and this can be avoided by drinking lots of fluids and sometimes even taking a mild stool softener. Foods such as figs, dates, plums, and prunes are natural laxatives. You can also try wheat bran cereal, pinto beans, bananas, apples, whole-grain breads, raw vegetables, and cashews. Drink plenty of water as well.

Sore mouth

The lining of the mouth has cells that normally divide and replace themselves frequently. Hence, like cancer cells, these cells are also affected by chemotherapy. Rarely, your mouth may become caked with a white lining. This is a **Candida** fungal infection (**thrush**), which can cause a sore mouth and difficulty swallowing. A special anti-fungal mouthwash will treat this. If your mouth is becoming dry from chemotherapy or drugs like antidepressants, make up a mouth wash with a mixture of warm salty water (a pinch of salt in a large glass of water is usually enough) and two pinches of baking soda. Sucking sugar-free lemon drops or chewing sugarless gum may help to stimulate your saliva.

Small mouth ulcers can occur about one week after chemotherapy is given and may last up to two weeks. These can be painful and can interfere with talking, drinking, and eating. If you have a lot of mouth ulcers, check with your doctor or nurse, because they can be a sign of or the cause of an infection requiring antibiotics in a hospital.

Avoid very hot or warm foods, and instead eat foods that are cold or at room temperature. If your mouth is sore, choose soothing foods such as mashed potatoes, pureed foods, scrambled eggs, macaroni and cheese, and custard. A small amount of ice cream may give you a much needed psychological boost and also sooth the mouth. Avoid irritating foods that contain acids, such as oranges, grapefruits, lemons, limes, very spicy or dry raw vegetables, and hard toasts and meats. Some patients experience a "metallic" taste and all foods may taste bland with certain chemotherapy drugs. Try using a variety of spices to restore taste to some foods while on chemotherapy, and avoid your favorite foods so that you can look forward to them when you gradually recover your taste when chemotherapy is complete.

You can suck on ice and chew sugarless gum, and you can moisten dry toast with some light margarine or some preserves. Also moisturize your lips with an unflavored and unmedicated lip balm or petroleum jelly.

Dental hygiene

It's a good idea for your dentist to check out your teeth and dental hygiene before you start chemotherapy, as occasionally chemotherapy can worsen a dental problem and cause a dental abscess. Choose a toothbrush with soft or extra-soft rounded bristles and soften them with warm water before you start brushing your teeth. It's best to use toothpaste with fluoride, which helps prevent cavities. Use dental floss or dental tape to clean between your teeth every day if possible. Toothpastes labeled "tartar control" help to get rid of the sticky film on your teeth that may speed up decay.

If you have had a problem with cracked fillings, check with your dentist to see if you grind your teeth at night. Grinding can also cause your jaw muscles to ache. Talk to your dentist about getting a specially fitted mouth guard to wear at night. Dental sensitivity can persist after chemotherapy is finished.

Menstrual periods and sexuality

Your periods may become irregular or stop entirely during chemotherapy. I'll go into more detail in the next chapter, but the bottom line is that if you are under the age of 35, there is a very high chance that your periods will come back within six months after chemotherapy. If you are aged 35 to 40, it's unpredictable, and if you are over 40 years of age, there is a reasonably high chance that you will lose all your ovarian function and not have periods again.

Every woman needs to go through menopause eventually. Unfortunately, with chemotherapy, you may go through it sooner rather than later. But look at the "good" effects of menopause: many of my patients are pleased that their periods have finally stopped and look forward to not needing contraception. More details about menstruation, fertility, menopause, and sexuality are given in Control Point #18 – Will Treatment Affect my Periods, Fertility, or Sex Life?

Fatigue

Fatigue is common and is a particular problem the week after your first course of chemotherapy. This can become worse as treatment goes on. Often, it is from lack of sleep. If necessary, ask for a sleeping pill, even if you have to take it once or twice a week just to catch up. Remember that it's like being in a war zone, going through all this treatment and stress.

Some good advice about improving your sleep is given at this web address:

www.helpguide.org/life/sleep_tips.htm

It is normal to feel tired and low, but remember that you will climb that mountain and see the light on the other side. This is a time to be kind to yourself and not over-commit to things you don't feel up to. Other causes of fatigue include a low blood count, particularly anemia; low thyroid hormone levels; heart disease; and sometimes even severe anxiety.

The National Cancer Institute has also produced some information on fatigue:

www.cancer.gov/cancertopics/pdq/supportivecare/fatigue/patient

Chemotherapy-induced nerve damage

Peripheral neuropathy is a common side effect of paclitaxel (Taxol) therapy. Typically, this occurs in the hands and feet as numbness and loss of coordination. Weekly rather than thrice-weekly doses cause fewer problems. Presenting symptoms include numbness, loss of the ability to differentiate hot from cold, and burning pain. Patients with a previous diagnosis of peripheral neuropathy or coexisting medical illnesses associated with peripheral neuropathy (such as diabetes mellitus or substantial prior alcohol use) appear to be especially prone to developing nerve damage. Research in preventing this side effect is ongoing. There is some experimental evidence that the antiepileptic drug gabapentin (Neurontin) may help, but clinical studies are continuing (Matsumoto 2006).

"Chemotherapy brain"

We don't really know what causes "**chemotherapy brain**" (the medical term is "cognitive changes"), but most women get through it, and it's usually only temporary. Hang in there; it usually gets better with time.

Memory problems can be due to a combination of going through menopause or to the chemotherapy itself. Estrogen receptors are located in areas of the brain related to memory, and the rapid decline in estrogen levels from chemotherapy or hormonal treatments probably are a big part of the problem.

Problems related to menopause tend to appear as problems with verbal memory (for example, not being able to find the correct word in a sentence or losing your thought mid-sentence) and sometimes visual memory (for example, difficulty with street signs or reading).

Chemotherapy-related memory dysfunction tends to manifest as problems with concentration, ability to focus, organization, and working with numbers. Many women feel forgetful and may struggle remembering people's names, remembering to do things, or learning new information.

Make sure you get a good night's sleep and consider taping important conversations or doctors' consultations. Stimulating the brain with exercise is important—try to keep reading and doing all the normal things to relax if possible.

Also reduce the amount of caffeine you drink and limit alcohol to no more than one glass a day. Make sure you have a task list and a notepad or diary at all times and write down all your appointments.

Weight gain

It is not uncommon to gain some weight during chemotherapy treatment. You may gain, on average, five to eight pounds (about two to four kilograms) while on chemotherapy. Weight gain may occur for a variety of reasons, including reduced activity, going through menopause, increased appetite, eating extra food and calories, and perhaps eating the wrong foods when you are feeling down. If this is the case and you want to stop gaining weight, here are some tips that can help, particularly after your chemotherapy is finished and you can get back to a normal routine. The National Cancer Institute (2003):

- Talk to a registered dietitian for more guidance

- Emphasize fruits, vegetables, and breads and cereals

- Choose lean meats (lean beef or pork trimmed of fat, chicken without skin) and low-fat dairy products (skim or 1% milk, light yogurt)

- Cut back on added butter, mayonnaise, sweets, and other extras

- Choose low-fat and low-calorie cooking methods (broiling, steaming)

- Avoid eating high-calorie snacks between meals

- If you feel up to it, increase the amount of exercise you get.

In the next chapter I will talk a lot more about the impact chemotherapy and hormonal treatments can have on your fertility and sexuality. These issues are really important and sometimes you will need to raise them with your health team as they are often overlooked.

CONTROL POINT #17 – DO I NEED CHEMOTHERAPY?

 WARNING Your white cells are at their lowest point two weeks after chemotherapy. If you get a fever, sweats, chills, a cough with yellow sputum, burning urine, a sore that won't heal, or diarrhea that won't settle down, call your doctor immediately so that antibiotics can be prescribed.

 TIP Having chemotherapy on a Friday gives you a couple of days when family is home on the weekend to help you recover, and you may be well enough to get back to work on Monday or Tuesday.

 REMEMBER The bigger your cancer, particularly if it's over 20 mm or there are lymph glands involved in your armpit, the greater the chance that chemotherapy will improve your prognosis.

Bec's Story

Knowing I was going to lose my hair was an enormous emotional challenge and strain. I was scared of how I would look, and what people would think. So, my hair began to fall out and my husband and children helped shave off what was left.

I took a nervous look in the mirror and felt a rush of strength capture me. I immediately knew I was not going to need a wig or scarf. Thoughts such as "I am stronger than the cancer ,and having lost my hair is no indication that I am not well" were racing through my mind.

From this day on I retained enormous strength within, helped by some very supporting comments from other cancer sufferers and people that I had met through my journey with breast cancer. Not feeling the need to cover my head gave me great strength in facing the survival of this illness.

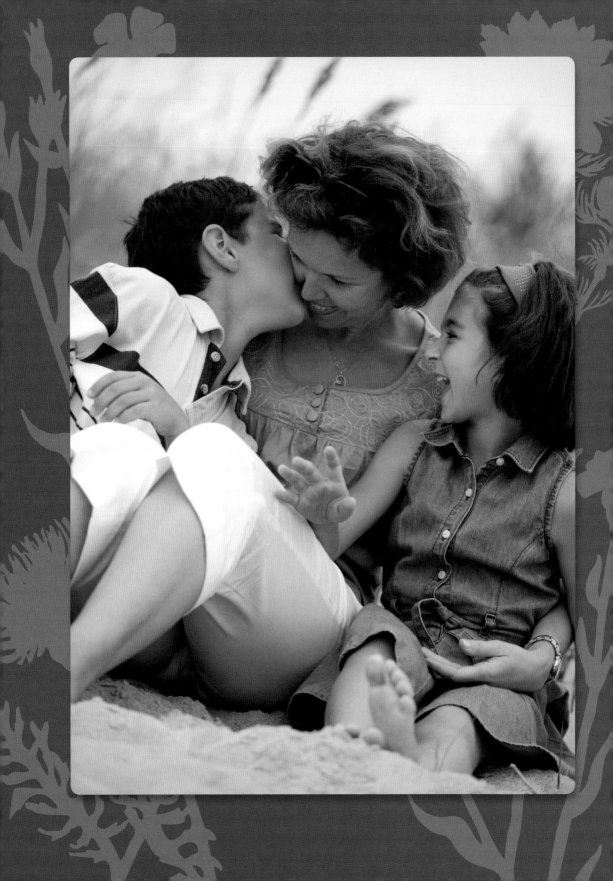

Control Point 18

Will Treatment Affect My Periods, Fertility, or Sex Life?

Control Point #18

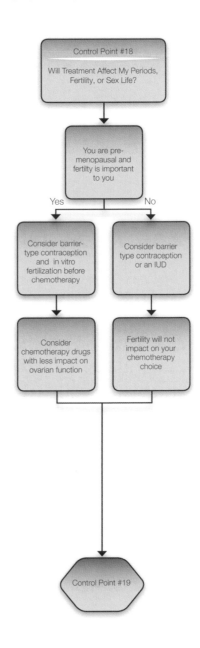

Control Point #18

Will Treatment Affect My Periods, Fertility, or Sex Life?

You are pre-menopausal and fertilty is important to you

Yes

No

Consider barrier-type contraception and in vitro fertilization before chemotherapy

Consider barrier type contraception or an IUD

Consider chemotherapy drugs with less impact on ovarian function

Fertility will not impact on your chemotherapy choice

Control Point #19

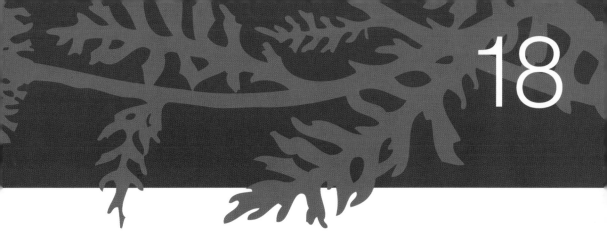

18

Will Treatment Affect My Periods, Fertility, or Sex Life?

More garden analogies

In my garden examples in the previous chapters, I mentioned that giving weed killer to the entire garden may inadvertently damage some normal plants. In many circumstances, the damage is temporary and the good plant can grow back and be totally normal. But sometimes the damage can be permanent. The ovary is one of those good plants that can be permanently affected by chemotherapy. Chemotherapy affects a woman's eggs, which are of course important for having babies, and the production of hormones in the ovaries, including estrogen. As mentioned in Control Point #11, many normal parts of the female body need estrogen to keep them healthy, including the breasts, vagina, heart, and bones.

There is a growing trend today, particularly in Western countries, to delay having children. This increases the number of women who have not yet started or completed their families when they are diagnosed with breast cancer. The bottom line is that if you are under the age of 35, there is a very high chance that your periods will come back within six months after chemotherapy. If you are aged 35 to 40, it's unpredictable, and if you are over 40, there is a reasonably high chance that you will lose all your ovarian function and have no more periods.

If you have not had any children and would like to in the future, it's really important to talk to your doctor about it as soon as possible, and if necessary see a fertility expert before your treatment starts.

Early menopause after treatment

It can be very distressing to find out that treatment may permanently cause early menopause and could thus affect your ability to have children. You may worry about how this could impact on a relationship if you have not had children with your current partner or if you do not have a partner. Discussing this can be a very difficult and delicate situation, particularly when it involves talking to a partner to whom you might never have spoken about the possibility of a long-term commitment.

It can also suddenly force a discussion about children and perhaps about going through the complexity of **in vitro fertilization** (IVF), when having children is the last thing on your mind. It's a little easier if your family is complete, although you may still experience a sense of loss. I remember having to counsel a woman I was treating, who already had a boy and a girl, but desperately wanted another child after her treatment. This was causing tension with her husband, who did not want any more children. Everyone is unique, so make sure your doctors and your partner know your true feelings.

The problem is that if you require chemotherapy, you may develop early menopause and become infertile because chemotherapy damages the eggs in your ovaries. Approximately one in four Western women under 50 years of age will experience menopause normally even without chemotherapy (McMahon 1966). As a rule of thumb, chemotherapy for breast cancer is said to add about ten years to ovarian age in terms of reproductive function (Hickey 2009). Goodwin (1999) found that use of either the first generation type of chemotherapy, called CMF, or the second generation type, called CEF, increased the risk of menopause for 40-year-old women to more than 40 percent. If you are a 50-year-old woman, the chance of going into menopause is close to 100 percent. If you are under 35 years of age, the chance of menopause is much lower: about 30% (Figure 90). Looking at Dr. Goodwin's data, it's clear that younger women tend to maintain their periods and do not generally become infertile.

I have treated many younger women with breast cancer and most have been able to have a baby after treatment if they wanted to. It feels very unfair being very young and having breast cancer. It is, of course, unfair at all ages, but for a young woman, there are additional issues that must be thought through, including:

- Trying to work and establish a career during treatment

- Maintaining or developing new relationships

- The issue of becoming infertile and losing the opportunity to have a family.

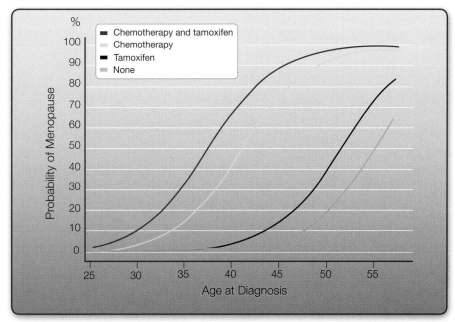

Figure 90: Estimated probability of menopause by age at diagnosis and type of treatment of breast cancer.

The timing of menstruation stopping

A second very important study involved several leading US cancer programs, including the Memorial Sloan-Kettering Cancer Center in New York and the University of Texas M.D. Anderson Cancer Center, Houston, which examined not only the chance of menstruation stopping with different types of chemotherapy but also when it stopped (Petrek 2006).

Figure 91 below shows the probability of your menstruation continuing after the commencement of chemotherapy. Of note is that the proportion of women with monthly bleeding dropped dramatically right after the first dose of chemotherapy. The percentage of the women with monthly bleeding reached a high of 55 percent 15 months after chemotherapy ended, but then gradually declined to a low of 35 percent five years after diagnosis.

Importantly, the US investigators found that women of all ages experienced problems with their menstrual function (Figure 92). However, most women aged 40 or older had no menstrual bleeding at the end of chemotherapy, and over a two to three year period, only one in five women, or 20 percent, kept menstruating.

In contrast, menstrual cycling recovered rapidly for women 35 years or younger; the proportion of women with bleeding rose to approximately 85 percent six months after the end of chemotherapy and remained relatively constant thereafter. If you are under 35 years of age, the chance of remaining fertile is high. However, remember that even

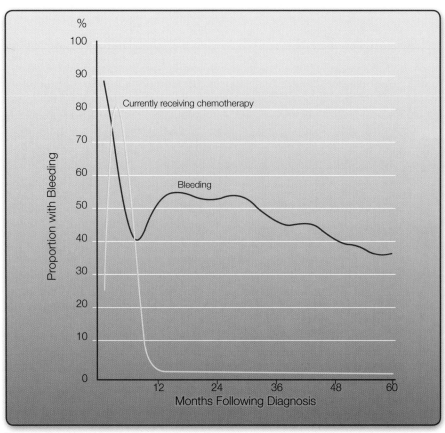

Figure 91: Probability of menstruation continuing by the number of months following the commencement of chemotherapy for breast cancer.

if your menstruation returns, you may still have an earlier menopause (and hence less time to become pregnant) than if you had never had chemotherapy. The recovery was less pronounced for women between the ages of 35 and 40, with a peak of about 60 percent experiencing monthly bleeding six months after the end of chemotherapy, and a low of 45 percent with bleeding at five years. If you are between 35 and 40 and wish to have children in the future, consider IVF and chemotherapy agents that may have a smaller chance of making you infertile (see next section).

The risk of early menopause by chemotherapy type

Figure 93 shows the chance of menstrual bleeding continuing after different types of chemotherapy given after your surgery. Two years after treatment, the chance of menstrual bleeding persisting was:

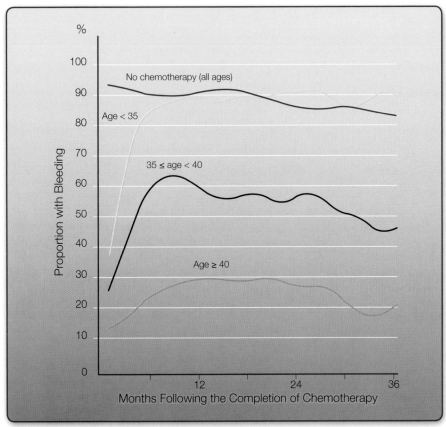

Figure 92: The probability of menstruation continuing following chemotherapy broken down by age at diagnosis of breast cancer.

No chemotherapy:	85%
AC: doxorubicin, cyclophosphamide:	60%
ACT: doxorubicin, cyclophosphamide, paclitaxel:	45%
TAC (or DAC): docetaxel, doxorubicin, cyclophosphamide:	40%
CMF: cyclophosphamide, methotrexate, fluorouracil:	30%

After any doxorubicin and cyclophosphamide (AC) regimen, there was a slow recovery phase of about nine months, followed by a plateau, during which almost half continued to bleed. In contrast, after CMF, there was no recovery phase and a continual decline in monthly bleeding, and only about one in five continued to bleed three years later. So, if retaining your fertility is important, the AC regimen may be a good compromise.

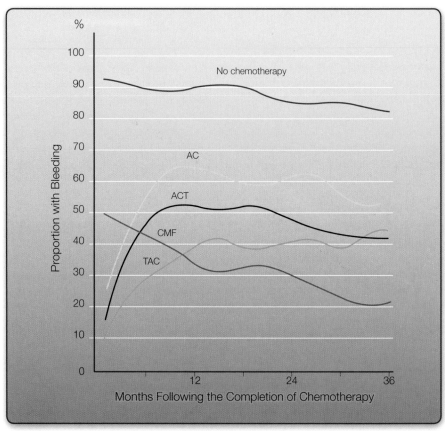

Figure 93: Chance of menstruation continuing over time by type of chemotherapy used.

I'd like to clarify two important points. Firstly, menopause is generally defined as the absence of menstruation for 12 months or more. This certainly applies if you have chemotherapy, but if you are on tamoxifen, it may be a "false menopause"; your periods can start again once you stop taking this medication. So just because your periods stop, particularly if it is within the first year of starting your chemotherapy or while on tamoxifen, do not assume that you no longer need contraception. Secondly, if your periods come back, it doesn't necessarily mean that you will still be fertile. If you cannot get pregnant after 12 months of trying, see a fertility expert.

Methods to preserve fertility

If you are very young and you have a partner, I often recommend IVF and freezing and storing embryos ("test tube babies") for possible later use. The American Society of Clinical Oncology published guidelines for doctors on this subject in 2006 (Lee 2006). It generally takes about two weeks to complete this step.

Starting on the second or third day of your period, you will start medications that will mature multiple eggs in your ovaries. You will have frequent blood tests and ovarian ultrasounds to monitor the development of your eggs.

After hormonal stimulation of your ovaries, the eggs are collected or "harvested" using a vaginal ultrasound while you're under a light anesthetic. These can then be fertilized in a test tube with sperm from your partner, or from a donor, depending on your own situation. IVF is done in the laboratory, not within your body. The fertilized eggs grow briefly into tiny embryos and are then frozen. When you're ready to have a baby, they can be thawed out and implanted into your womb (uterus).

The second approach, which is being tested around the world, is egg freezing, where a piece of your ovary is frozen and then later implanted back into your body. There have been very few babies born worldwide following this procedure, so I wouldn't guarantee it, and it's likely to be expensive.

Another technique that you may want to use if you do not have a partner is suppressing the ovary with drugs such as Zoladex, given about one week before your chemotherapy starts and until three weeks after the last chemotherapy dose. This is quite a simple technique and worth considering, but please talk to your doctor about this much-debated method.

You may wish to talk to someone who has been through a similar cancer experience. Every state in Australia, for example, offers Cancer Connect, linking people over the phone who have been through similar cancer experiences by calling 13 11 20. In the US, a useful website is Fertile Hope, found at www.fertilehope.org/.

RESOLVE is another organization that provides education and support to individuals with fertility problems in the US. For information, go to www.resolve.org or a website for young women's cancer, www.youngsurvival.org.

I can't go into all the ethical issues involved in this field. There are some heart-wrenching decisions that need to be made. Having to deal with these issues with a new partner when you have never even discussed marriage, let alone pregnancy, is difficult to say the least. Concerns about passing on a breast cancer gene to the next generation need to be discussed with your doctor too, and obviously all the ethical and emotional issues associated with donor sperm need fairly rapid discussion and thinking through before you start your chemotherapy.

Contraception after breast cancer

Conventional wisdom is to stop "the pill" or other hormonal contraception after being diagnosed with breast cancer. This may mean you need to use alternative contraception that may have implications for your relationship. If you're having chemotherapy, just because your periods have stopped doesn't mean that you've become infertile. Take care and continue to use barrier contraception (such as condoms or a diaphragm with spermicide) or intrauterine devices (IUDs). Some, but not all oncologists recommend an IUD that releases a small amount of a man-made hormone into your womb every day. If your tumor is estrogen receptor-negative, doing so is unlikely to cause any harm.

If you are taking tamoxifen, take extra care to avoid pregnancy. Tamoxifen use increases the chance of menstruation stopping even more than chemotherapy does. The highest chance of menstruation stopping occurs if you have both chemotherapy and tamoxifen (Figure 90). However, the mechanism by which it does this is different and potentially reversible. Tamoxifen can also stimulate ovulation, so don't rely on it as a contraceptive.

So, if you are taking tamoxifen and your periods stop, you may still be fertile, and you should use barrier-type contraception or an IUD. Further, if you are under the age of 50 and your periods have stopped while on tamoxifen, it's best not to take one of the AIs (aromatase inhibitors; e.g., anastrozole, letrozole or exemestane) mentioned earlier, because they may in fact stimulate your ovaries to produce an egg (ovulation) and cause an unwanted pregnancy (Mourits 2007, Smith 2006).

Having a baby after breast cancer

A difficult and emotional issue to face is becoming pregnant after breast cancer. Important issues for discussion include whether or not the pregnancy can cause harm from the associated increased estrogen levels. There have been a few case reports of problems, but most large studies have not shown an adverse effect on your prognosis from pregnancy after breast cancer. What about the timing of pregnancy? While many doctors advise waiting two years after treatment, there is no science to this whatsoever, and I have had many patients have children as early as six months after all treatment stops. It depends on factors such as your current age and the chances of your breast cancer coming back. Even if your periods have returned, your chances of becoming pregnant may not be as high as they were before your breast cancer treatment. One important aspect to consider, as I noted above, is that you may reach menopause earlier than you would have if you hadn't had breast cancer.

If you are on tamoxifen, I suggest stopping it for at least two to three months before you try to get pregnant to ensure that it's totally out of your system. It's best to talk to your doctor about starting tamoxifen again after you have finished breastfeeding. If you have become pregnant while on tamoxifen, discuss this with your oncologist and obstetrician as soon as possible. The chance of damage to the baby is very low, but there have been a few case reports of malformations (Berger 2008).

The hardest aspect of all this, though, is the awful thought of how you and your partner could look after yourself and a baby if by chance the cancer comes back or, in the worst case, you don't survive your breast cancer. If you have good family support and feel that your partner could look after a child even if you were not around, then there is no reason to avoid the pleasure of having a child.

It's certainly not an easy choice to make, though. If I see a patient who wants to have a child after a previous diagnosis of breast cancer, it generally is quite a long consultation. I discuss factors such as:

- Prognosis
- Partner and family support if you do get breast cancer again during your pregnancy or after you have a baby
- The fact that becoming pregnant doesn't seem to make your prognosis worse
- Breastfeeding, which is not possible on the treated side
- The fact that your normal breast enlarges during pregnancy, while your breast treated by lumpectomy and radiation doesn't change size or produce milk, which can result in an imbalance
- The role of tests: I normally recommend a CT scan of your body and a bone scan to be quite sure there is no sign of cancer before you get pregnant. I also organize a mammogram and ultrasound, as it's impossible to see through the normal breast once you start breastfeeding
- The fact that the incidence of miscarriage or fetal abnormalities following treatment is not increased (Durrieu 2004, Kroman 1997).

If you can't get pregnant, you may have to look at more difficult pathways, such as national or international adoption. Many agencies are not supportive of women with breast cancer adopting babies, but speak to your doctor about a letter of support.

Coping with menopause

Menopause symptoms after breast cancer treatments

Symptoms of menopause are the most frequent and troublesome side effect after treatment of breast cancer with chemotherapy or hormonal treatment. It's one of the most common concerns I discuss with my patients after their treatment. Many go through menopause without any problems at all, whereas others have a tough time with severe hot flashes and night sweats.

Usually your body can adjust to reduced estrogen, and many of these symptoms will improve on their own over time. It's hard at first when estrogen levels drop suddenly after treatment rather than gradually over time, as they would with a natural menopause. Common symptoms from reduced levels of estrogen in your body can be classified as follows:

Vasomotor

- Hot flashes and night sweats are common. They can be mild (occurring once or twice a day) or severe (more than 20 per day)

- Heart palpitations or

- Headaches.

Sexual

- Vaginal dryness and pain with intercourse are more typically problems with aromatase inhibitors, but they can occur after tamoxifen or from a chemotherapy-induced menopause

- Urinary frequency and occasional stress incontinence are not uncommon

- Reduced sex drive is quite common, particularly during treatment.

Psychological

- Feeling down, tired, anxious, or irritable can be caused by menopause, particularly while you are feeling pressured during treatment

- Poor sleep can be a direct side effect of hormonal treatments, particularly aromatase inhibitors, but is also secondary to menopause

- Poor memory and concentration may be a direct menopausal effect, or more likely may be related to sleep deprivation or a direct effect of hormonal treatments, based on a few small studies.

Somatic or Physical

- Bone thinning (see Control Point 16). Consider taking calcium, vitamin D, or using a bisphosphonate if you have established bone thinning or loss. For example, zoledronic acid (Zometa) 4 mg intravenously every six months effectively inhibited bone loss for patients on aromatase inhibitors, Zoladex, and even tamoxifen (Chien 2006)

- Joint aches can occur and are best managed with stretching, exercise, and glucosamine. Sometimes anti-arthritis tablets can help. In severe cases with an AI, it may be best to switch to tamoxifen or stop the drug altogether (Felson 2005).

- Dry skin or a sensation of ants crawling under your skin ("formication"). This usually goes away on its own with time. Use a regular moisturizer even if it does get better.

Possible treatments to help menopause symptoms

- Many things can aggravate hot flashes, including stress, hot drinks, alcohol (particularly red wine), overheating the body in spas or baths, hot weather, and spicy foods. Both negative stress and positive stress (such as a party) can aggravate hot flashes. Avoiding these factors can help. Paced breathing with deep inhalations, holding for five seconds and then breathing out slowly, can help. This is a good way to relax. Find a quiet room and put on some calming music and do this for about ten to 15 minutes a day in one or two sessions. Relaxation techniques such as yoga or massage can help too. A Finnish study found that traditional Chinese acupuncture may be helpful, and a Chillow® pillow can also help. See www.chillow.co.uk. Wearing clothes made from natural fabrics such as cotton, silk, or linen in layers that you can take on or off as you get hot or cold is also practical.

- Use of non-hormonal herbal therapies or vitamins such as Remifemin (an extract of black cohosh)(two tablets morning and night), a red clover extract such as Promensil (one tablet a day), or vitamin E (800 international units [IU] per day) can sometimes help with mild hot flashes and night sweats. Always read the instructions and precautions before you take these over-the-counter drugs; just because they are not prescription does not mean they cannot be dangerous if misused. Several case reports of possible severe liver damage have been reported with black cohosh (and therefore it is not available in all countries), but millions of people use this every year so the risk is extremely low. Another alternative for mild symptoms is low dose clonidine (Catapres). The initial oral dose for hot flash treatment is 0.05 mg twice daily, but you may require at least 0.1 mg twice daily. The clonidine patch, delivering 0.1 mg/day, can also be considered, but it is not available in some countries. When discontinuing higher dose therapy, gradually decrease the dose rather than stopping it suddenly. Clonidine has been used in higher doses for blood pressure control, but it can cause side effects, such as dry mouth, constipation, drowsiness, or difficulty sleeping.

- If the hot flashes continue or are moderately severe, the same drugs used to treat anxiety and depression, such as venlafaxine (Efexor), can be helpful in lower doses. The starting dose is 37.5 mg daily for two weeks and then 75 mg daily. If it doesn't help within four weeks, it's best to try something else. I tend to start with this medicine if your symptoms are moderately severe (for example, more than ten hot flashes or episodes of night sweats a day) or if you have significant psychological effects or difficulty sleeping. Venlafaxine can cause weight loss by causing loss of appetite, and may be preferred by overweight women for this reason. Reduced libido and difficulty achieving orgasm has been reported in about one in five women taking this drug for anxiety or depression (Kennedy 2000).

- Another drug in this class of medicines is paroxetine (Paxil), with a starting dose of 10 mg daily increasing to 20 mg daily after one to two weeks. It is best, however, not to take paroxetine if you are on tamoxifen, as paroxetine can make tamoxifen less effective by breaking down its active ingredient. Side effects, especially nausea and reduced libido, should be monitored. Reduced libido and difficulty achieving orgasm has been reported in about one in two women taking this drug for anxiety or depression (Kennedy 2000). A few case reports of increased libido have also been reported (Pae 2005). Paroxetine is best taken at night because it sometimes causes drowsiness. Paroxetine has similar side effects to venlafaxine, although less nausea and anorexia. It can also rarely cause blurred vision.

- Some doctors try other drugs, such as gabapentin (Neurontin) (up to 300 mg three times a day), which is used for nerve pain. I tend to start patients on a dose of 100 mg per day, to be taken at bedtime particularly if you're over 65, as it can cause dizziness. If you continue to have hot flashes, the dose can be increased to 300 mg twice daily and then to three times daily, at two-week intervals. Antacids for heartburn can reduce the effectiveness of gabapentin, which should be taken at least two hours after antacid use.

- If all else fails, some form of short-term hormone replacement therapy (HRT) may be needed. Progesterone tablets, such as low doses of Provera or Megace, are very effective in treating night sweats but are probably not safe to take for long periods because of their link to causing breast cancer when taken as a form of HRT with estrogen. However, a counter argument is that we used high doses of Provera as a form of treatment of breast cancer for many years in the 80s. Certainly, if your tumor is ER-negative, it's probably safe as a short-term measure. If progesterone tablets fail, HRT such as tibolone (Livial), available in the UK and Australia, appears to be safe for women with ER-negative breast cancer, but a recent study has found that it increases the risk of cancer coming back if the original breast cancer was ER-positive (Kenemans 2009). The problem with the study was that the number of patients in the study was small, so we can't be too sure of the statistics just yet. In the US, low-dose estrogen therapy, or estrogen and progestogen HRT, may be considered for severe symptoms of menopause, but you need to be aware that this may increase the chance of your cancer coming back.

- Vaginal estrogen can help with dryness and reduced vaginal tone, but it's probably best avoided if you're taking an aromatase inhibitor because, theoretically, the small amount of vaginal absorption may counteract the effect of the AI (Kendall 2006). Although many oncologists are reluctant to use vaginal estrogens with an AI, their use was allowed in the large MA-17 trial, which examined five years of letrozole after five years of tamoxifen without adverse effects reported (Goss 2005).

- Use water-based vaginal lubricants and moisturizers. Vaginal moisturizers such as vitamin E or Replens should be used on a regular basis after you shower to help hydrate and revitalize the vaginal lining and vulva. Lubricants should be used liberally during intercourse. Krychman (2009) has advised that lubricants, especially those without flavors, colors, or warming additives, can and should be used during intercourse. He also notes that lubricants like Vaseline and oil-based products should be avoided since they can change the natural balance of vaginal bacteria and in some women may lead to infections. Excellent lubricants include Slippery Stuff and Sylk. Care should be used with Astroglide and KY Jelly, as some women find these products drying and the additives in them may be irritating.

There is no right answer and you need to balance your symptoms with the possible side effects and risks of taking some of these countermeasures. The evidence one way or the other is weak to say the least, so "Taking Control" here means understanding your options, talking to your treatment team, and seeing an understanding gynecologist if required for an examination and advice.

Impact of treatment on sexuality

The diagnosis of breast cancer can affect the way you view yourself and your sexuality. Sexuality is often not discussed by doctors who may be concerned that doing so will extend the length of their consultation or who may just feel uncomfortable talking about the subject. Some health professionals equate sex only with intercourse, which of course is only one facet of human sexuality. Most of my patients do suffer at least a temporary reduction in sex drive and intimacy, and there is no doubt that this can put pressure on relationships. Often there is an enormous loss of self-esteem following the loss of a breast, which is only partially helped by a reconstruction. A mastectomy can have different effects on different people. I've treated some patients who are comfortable lying topless on the beach after a mastectomy, whereas most feel a loss of self-esteem and become self-conscious about being seen nude. What I often observe is that women are more worried than their partner about losing their breast.

On the other hand, women who have breast conservation tend to feel more positive about their body image but may sometimes be left with an underlying sense of concern about cancer coming back in the breast that is left behind. Women who have breast conservation often do not appreciate their treated breast being caressed, particularly in the first year or two after treatment, because of increased tenderness and swelling. Nipple sensitivity can also be reduced temporarily or permanently after treatment.

The most common problem I see with my patients is just "feeling awful" during chemotherapy—the loss of your hair, gaining weight, feeling sick, feeling tired, managing hot flashes and dropping levels of estrogen combined with the physical effects of surgery make women turn off sexually. No wonder you're not feeling sexy. Sometimes, the loss of libido is temporary or has already been occurring for some time. If it persists, speak to your doctor or ask for a referral to an expert in this field. It's often hard to bring this topic up with your health professional, but you'll be glad you did. You can talk to a breast care nurse if available or try these questions or statements:

- I'm having problems with my relationship with my partner

- I have vaginal dryness that is making sex less enjoyable

- My sex drive has gone down or I have lost interest in sex

- What vaginal lubricants can I use?

- What are the symptoms associated with menopause?

- What should I do about contraception?

You have a right to information and non-judgmental care. If you are not satisfied, ask for a second opinion from a relationship or sexual health expert.

As mentioned in the chapter on hormonal treatments, drugs such as aromatase inhibitors (AIs) can also cause side effects such as weight gain, tiredness, and sleeplessness, which can indirectly affect sex drive and self-esteem. Further, AIs can cause loss of libido, difficulty achieving orgasm, or total loss of orgasm. In such cases, I usually switch my patients to tamoxifen, which has less impact on sexuality.

I'm not a big fan of testosterone tablets or cream to try to increase sex drive, as this can be converted to estrogen in the body and theoretically make matters worse. As mentioned above, sometimes drugs like venlafaxine (Efexor) or paroxetine (Paxil) that used to help hot flashes can cause loss of orgasm. It's very important to work out the timing of your loss of orgasm with any new medications you may have been given.

Another factor that can impact on sexuality is just feeling down, both during and after all your treatment. It is very normal to feel flat, sad, crushed, knocked down, sleep deprived, disorganized, or even feel that things are hopeless, but most people most times will just work these through and come out stronger and better equipped, usually without needing antidepressants along the way. Try to avoid antidepressants as a "quick fix," and instead seek to normalize your sleep patterns, become more active, organize "dates" with your partner, and schedule some regular activities such as going to the movies, meeting up with friends, or starting a regular walking group with your neighbors. If you have problems getting to sleep, waking up early and not being able to go back to sleep, or just feel lousy and less motivated to do your normal routine, seek advice from your family doctor. Here are some ideas:

- Keep communicating about sex and intimacy

- Use water-based vaginal lubricants during sex

- Don't always have intercourse. External closeness, or "outercourse," is a good alternative, particularly as you start recovering from treatment

- Attend a *Look Good Feel Better* workshop and wear some makeup if you enjoy the way it makes you look and feel

- For partners, give your loved one a head-to-toe massage, which will help her relax and build up her self-esteem and will be much appreciated

- If you don't feel like sex, try to give your partner a massage and/or bring him or her to orgasm without intercourse

- Take short breaks away, preferably without the children

- Speak to your doctor about using vaginal estrogen if vaginal dryness is causing pain with intercourse

- Exercise at least three times a week

- If you have a sudden loss of sex drive and orgasm, check with your doctor about whether it could be treatment related

- After treatment, look at buying some new sexy lingerie and see a specialist bra fitter who is experienced with women who have had breast cancer

- Dye your hair if it comes back grayer after chemotherapy

- See a sex therapist if you are concerned about your situation

- And just to reiterate, keep talking to your partner; they will have their ups and downs too, and may feel lost and scared about the thought of losing you

- Tell your partner that you will get through your treatment and life will get back to some new normality where you can spend some time together deciding new priorities for yourselves, your relationship, and your lifestyle

- See www.breastcancer.org/tips/intimacy/

Remember, your partner loves you because of you, not because of your breast. An important step is to show your partner the new you after your surgery. It's never easy at first. Most men do cope, but many can't communicate as well as you and need some prompting. Many relationships become strengthened after breast cancer; but sadly, a few fall apart. If you are not in a relationship, finding a suitable and available companion is always a challenge—with or without breast cancer (se Silvana's story). I've seen many, many success stories of women meeting new partners after breast cancer. Connecting and becoming friends is important in any relationship. When trust has been established, letting them know about your condition and what you have been through is very important. Be honest and put the issue "on the table." If they can't cope with it, you don't want to know them anyway and deserve much better.

CONTROL POINT #18 – WILL TREATMENT AFFECT MY PERIODS, FERTILITY, OR SEX LIFE?

 WARNING If you are roughly 45 to 50 years of age, your periods have stopped from chemotherapy, and you need hormonal treatment, it may be best to consider tamoxifen rather than an aromatase inhibitor first until you know for certain that your periods won't come back. Aromatase inhibitors can sometimes stimulate the production of eggs in your ovaries and cause an unexpected pregnancy if you haven't actually gone into menopause.

 TIP The younger you are, particularly if you're under 35, the less likely that chemotherapy or hormonal treatment will make you infertile. Use water-based lubricants when you have sex and use a vaginal moisturizer regularly after your shower.

 REMEMBER It's best to stop all hormonal contraception after being diagnosed with breast cancer, and therefore sexuality may become a problem. Talk to your doctors and nurses about your options for contraception. Communicate with your partner about sexuality and intimacy.

Silvana's Story

Learning that I had cancer, and then losing a breast was hard, especially as I had recently separated from my husband. But hitting the dating scene again was something I hadn't even considered. I mean, how do you tell someone that you only have one breast? And when is the best time to tell them?

I know there are many guys out there who would run a mile with the thought that the girl they are seeing is 'deformed'. When I decided to start dating again, I wasn't really thinking about the intimacy part and was more focused on finding someone I was interested in, who would also be interested in me.

I put my name down on one of the matchmaking websites, and at the same time had a friend suggest emailing someone they knew, so before long I was corresponding with a handful of different people. The mutual friend intrigued me. He seemed to be able to just put the right words down every time. I commented that my photo was of me with very short hair because it was growing back from chemo, and waited for the reaction.

I expected the interest to drop immediately, however was very surprised when he responded that this meant I was a battler, and that was a good thing. We met, and he asked what sort of cancer I had. I told him that it was breast cancer and that I was indeed lopsided. Did he run away? Not in the least.

He smiled, and said he had seen plenty of scars. I know that the man I met is most unusual, and that many men would have turned tail. But I also know that if I hadn't taken the step to look I would never have found him, and I can truly say that he is the best thing that has happened to me for a very long time.

I didn't know what I was looking for, or that I needed a man who understands the depth of change a person goes through with cancer, someone with a degree of empathy and understanding. I was fortunate to find someone just like that.

If you keep in your mind that life is a journey, then make the most of your journey and explore all of your options. Don't narrow down your life and be tied to the fact that you are 'different'. Find a man who appreciates someone who is not the same as all the rest.

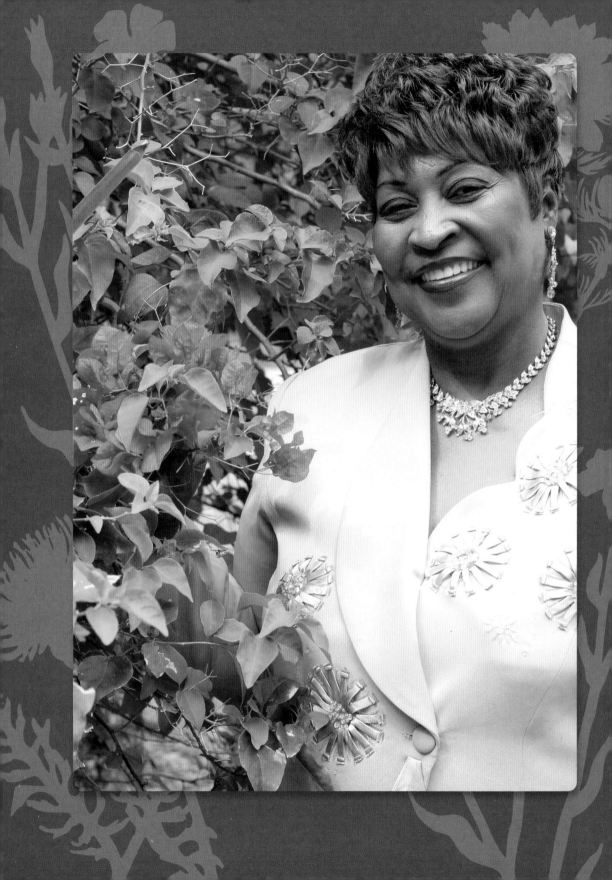

Control Point 19

Do I Need Herceptin (Trastuzumab)?

Control Point #19

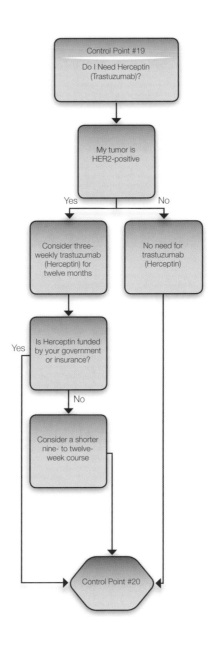

Control Point #19

Do I Need Herceptin (Trastuzumab)?

My tumor is HER2-positive

Yes → Consider three-weekly trastuzumab (Herceptin) for twelve months

No → No need for trastuzumab (Herceptin)

Is Herceptin funded by your government or insurance?

Yes →

No → Consider a shorter nine- to twelve-week course

Control Point #20

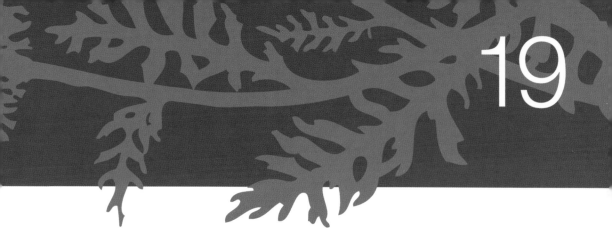

Do I Need Herceptin (Trastuzumab)?

What is Herceptin?

Herceptin is a targeted treatment for breast cancer. A lot of our conventional treatments, like chemotherapy, have to treat normal and abnormal cells. Herceptin is less like a "scatter gun" and more like a "sniper gun." It locks onto or "intercepts" its target without causing a lot of damage elsewhere.

As mentioned in my weed example above, giving chemotherapy is like using weed killer that can kill off the weed but also damage the normal plants and grass. Using targeted treatments like Herceptin is like giving a very specific weed killer that, for example, kills off clover in your grass but leaves your grass untouched.

Herceptin is what's called a **monoclonal antibody**, and it's biological targeted cancer treatment. Antibodies are molecules made naturally by our immune systems, and monoclonal ones are manufactured in the lab. Herceptin targets breast cancer cells that have a particular target called the HER2 receptor. You may also hear Herceptin called trastuzumab. This is its generic name, and Herceptin is the more popular brand name. Herceptin also increases the effect of chemotherapy drugs on breast cancer cells.

A book about Dr. Slamon's discovery of Herceptin, was made into a television filmcalled Living Proof in 2008 starring Harry Connick, Jr. It's worth watching.

What is the HER2 receptor?

The American Association for Cancer Research (AACR) gives some good information about the HER2 gene on their website:

www.aacr.org/home/public--media/patients--family/fact-sheets/cancer-concepts/her2.aspx

The HER2 (human epidermal growth factor receptor 2) gene is part of a family of genes that play roles in regulating cell growth.

About 20 out of every 100 patients with breast cancer have a large amount of the HER2 protein on the surface of their breast cancer cells. This is called HER2-positive breast cancer and is shown in Figure 94 in green. This protein is called a growth factor receptor because it transmits signals from growth factors outside of cells to the inside. These signals make the cells grow properly only when there is the correct number of receptors on the cell surface.

Testing for the receptor was described earlier (see the HER2 receptor) and can take up to two weeks for the absolute final test (called the "ISH" test) to come back. It's uncommon for women with invasive lobular or grade 1 invasive ductal carcinomas to be HER2-positive. Don't get too worried if you're HER2-negative; it's good news because your tumor is probably less aggressive than an HER2-positive tumor. If your tumor is HER2-positive, that's also good news because you can have Herceptin.

The excess number of HER2 receptors on the cell surface for women with HER2-positive breast cancer can result in unregulated cell growth. Tumors that are HER2-positive appear to be faster growing and may be less sensitive to some types of chemotherapy and hormonal treatment.

The Herceptin antibody (shown in yellow) or drug attaches itself to this protein receptor and blocks it so that the growth factors can no longer tell the cancer cells to grow. There are new drugs against the HER2 receptor being developed all the time, and new trials for testing them.

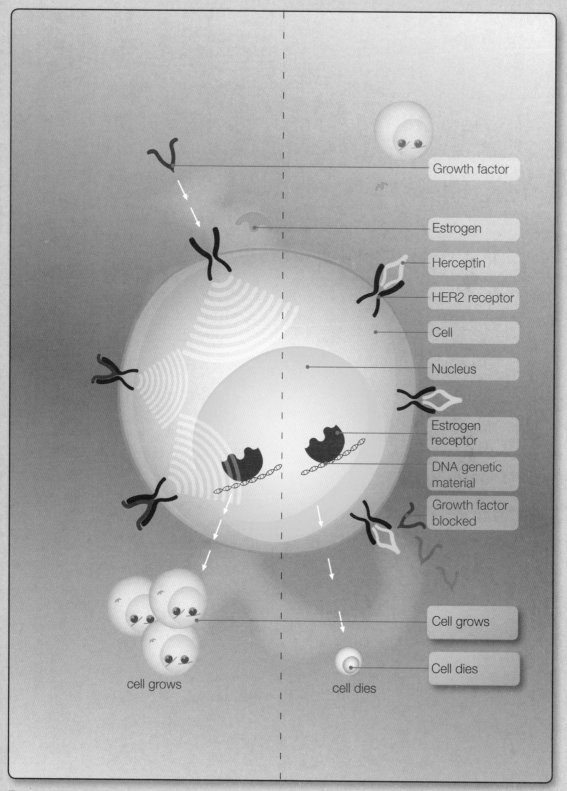

Growth factor

Estrogen

Herceptin

HER2 receptor

Cell

Nucleus

Estrogen receptor

DNA genetic material

Growth factor blocked

Cell grows

Cell dies

cell grows

cell dies

Figure 94: HER2 receptors (green) are stimulated by growth factors (red) and can be blocked by trastuzumab (Herceptin) (yellow).

Who can have Herceptin?

Government guidelines vary. In some countries, because of the cost, it can only be used if the cancer has already spread (too little too late, in my opinion). Many countries, including Australia, the UK and New Zealand recommend and publicly fund Herceptin for up to one year for all patients with early stage HER2 positive breast cancer irrespective of whether or not the cancer has spread to the lymph glands.

What is the evidence that Herceptin works?

Herceptin was first proven to work for women whose cancer had spread to other parts of their body. In 2005, the results of four clinical trials showed that Herceptin was also effective in the treatment of HER2-positive breast cancer that had not spread. Women who received Herceptin and chemotherapy lived longer and had significantly less chance of the breast cancer coming back than women who received chemotherapy without Herceptin. An analysis of the first two large clinical trials, with over 3,500 patients, showed that women on Herceptin had almost a 91 percent chance of survival four years after diagnosis and women who had chemotherapy only had an 86 percent chance (Romond 2005). This is quite a big difference.

Another study that really impressed me had to be stopped early because of the clear effectiveness of one course of treatment. In that study, patients with very large, HER2-positive, operable breast cancers were randomly assigned to either four cycles of paclitaxel followed by four cycles of FEC chemotherapy, or to the same chemotherapy with simultaneous weekly Herceptin for 24 weeks (Buzdar 2005). After 34 patients had completed therapy, the trial's data monitoring committee stopped the trial because of the marked superiority of Herceptin plus chemotherapy. Complete disappearance of cancer following surgery occurred in 25 percent of women who did not receive Herceptin, and in 67 percent who did receive it! Such high rates of remission had not been seen before for patients with large breast cancers having only chemotherapy.

Dr. Dennis Slamon, the scientist who laid the groundwork for the development of Herceptin, recently showed that using a chemotherapy combination that eliminated Adriamycin but used Taxotere and an older drug called carboplatin, along with one year of Herceptin (TCp-H), had equivalent survival rates to conventional regimens with less impact on the heart and no risk of leukemia (Robert 2007).

How is Herceptin given?

You take Herceptin through a drip into a vein in your arm or into one of the main veins in the chest area or upper arm via a port. It takes about 30–60 minutes each time. Trials have looked into the best way to give Herceptin. Although it was initially given on a weekly basis, three weekly treatments appear to be just as good and definitely more convenient. Herceptin is sometimes given with chemotherapy, sometimes after chemotherapy, and sometimes on its own. Herceptin can be given safely with radiation and does not increase its side effects (Halyard 2006). How it is used depends on many factors, such as the fitness of the woman, the type of chemotherapy she is using, and what treatments she has used before.

What are the side effects of Herceptin?

The most talked about side effect is heart problems. If you are suitable for Herceptin, you will have tests on your heart before you start treatment and usually every three months throughout your course of treatment. If there is any sign that Herceptin is causing heart problems, your doctor may recommend that you stop the treatment. The heart can be checked in different ways: a CT scan, a nuclear study (a "gated heart pool scan"), or an echocardiogram (a type of ultrasound of the heart, also known as an "echo"). The echo is advantageous because it's quick and avoids radiation. Other common side effects are fatigue; diarrhea; and flu-like symptoms such as fevers,aches, and pains. These side effects tend to get less severe after the first course of treatment. Herceptin does not cause hair loss, which is a real bonus.

For how long is Herceptin given?

Nobody really knows the best duration of treatment and trials are still underway. Most of the reported trials gave 12 to 24 months of Herceptin. A Finnish study found that nine weeks of Herceptin was also beneficial, and this is probably a good option if you need to pay for Herceptin yourself (Joensuu 2006, 2009). The standard duration of treatment for Herceptin is 12 months (Goldhirsch 2009).

What's the bottom line about Herceptin?

My view about Herceptin is as follows:

- It looks like a good drug, particularly if you have higher risk breast cancer that has spread to the lymph glands

- Be cautious with it if you have heart disease, and get a heart scan at least every third course, particularly if you are having chemotherapy

- The long-term benefit is not known, but the early results look promising

- The standard duration of treatment is 12 months and it seems to be more effective when combined with chemotherapy

- If you can't afford it, don't panic; the success rates without it can still be high. Remember, in the largest trial (the combined trial above), the difference in recurrence rates between the treated and the untreated group was only 5 percent.

- Consider having the short "nine-week" Finnish variety of treatment as a minimum if you are HER2-positive and do not have insurance or access to government-funded Herceptin

- At this stage, there are mixed results about the benefit of Herceptin for women with smaller, good-prognosis tumors that are HER2-positive, but it is likely to have a benefit in this group of patients

- Most recurrences for patients with HER2-positive tumors tend to happen in the first five years. It may be that HER2 is a predictor of early relapse (similar to ER-negative and grade 3 tumors), rather than being an adverse factor all the time.

- Some, but not all, studies have found that patients with HER2-positive tumors have a higher risk of relapse in the brain. If you are having a CT scan for any reason, it only takes a few extra minutes to scan the brain as well.

- You can have Herceptin while you are having radiation therapy or chemotherapy

- The long-term side effects from Herceptin are not really known, but toxicity is slightly less if Adriamycin is not given.

What's in the pipeline?

There are always new drugs in the pipeline. See if your doctor has access to any new clinical trials. Another drug is lapatinib, which works for HER2-positive patients in a different and perhaps complementary way to Herceptin.

Stimulation of the HER2 receptor activates something called a tyrosine kinase enzyme inside the cell, which can prompt the cancer cell to grow. Specific drugs have been developed to stop (or inhibit) the enzyme, and therefore stop the growth factor receptor from activating the cancer cell. These drugs are known as **tyrosine kinase inhibitors** (TKIs). Lapatinib is also known as Tykerb.

The advantage of lapatinib is that it's a tablet that can be taken an hour before or after food. It's usually taken for advanced breast cancer with a chemotherapy tablet called Xeloda or capecitabine (Geyer 2006).

Trials are now testing Herceptin with or without lapatinib before surgery, and laboratory evidence suggests that giving the two together may be better than either alone. The most common side effects are acne, diarrhea, tiredness, and nausea.

It's likely that once all the trials for drugs such as lapatinib, and other newer drugs like **Avastin** (bevacizumab), are completed on patients with advanced breast cancer, they may turn out to be useful for patients with breast cancer still confined to the breast and lymph glands as well. Avastin is a monoclonal antibody against vascular endothelial growth factor-A (VEGF-A), which inhibits tumor growth by blocking the formation of new blood vessels (angiogenesis) that feed the cancer. There are some ongoing studies of Avastin for patients with triple-negative breast cancer often being combined with drugs like cisplatin, an old-fashioned agent we first used for patients with ovarian or testicular cancer that appears to be effective.

Another area that is of real interest now in the laboratory and the clinic are new drugs called poly (ADP-ribose) polymerase ("PARP") inhibitors. These drugs prevent the repair of DNA specifically in breast cancer cells causing them to die off, particularly for women who have the breast cancer gene, who often have "triple-negative" or "basal type" breast cancer. Ixabepilone is also a new drug that shows promise for triple-negative breast cancer (Baselga 2009).

The great news is that there are more and more new agents being tested that seem to hit the breast cancer cells more and the normal cells less. In the near future, treatment will become increasingly personalized, based on testing of your own metabolism, genetic profile, and specific receptors of your breast cancer cells.

CONTROL POINT #19 – DO I NEED HERCEPTIN (TRASTUZUMAB)?

WARNING You will have heart tests throughout your treatment course—one about every three months. Common side effects are fatigue; diarrhea; and flu-like symptoms such as fevers, aches, and pains. These side effects tend to get less severe after the first course of treatment.

TIP Don't get too worried if you're HER2-negative; it's good news because your tumor is probably less aggressive than an HER2-positive tumor. If your tumor is HER2-positive, treatment with Herceptin is very beneficial.

REMEMBER Herceptin is only effective in about one in five women who have cancers that are HER2-positive, does not cause hair loss and can be given with radiation or chemotherapy.

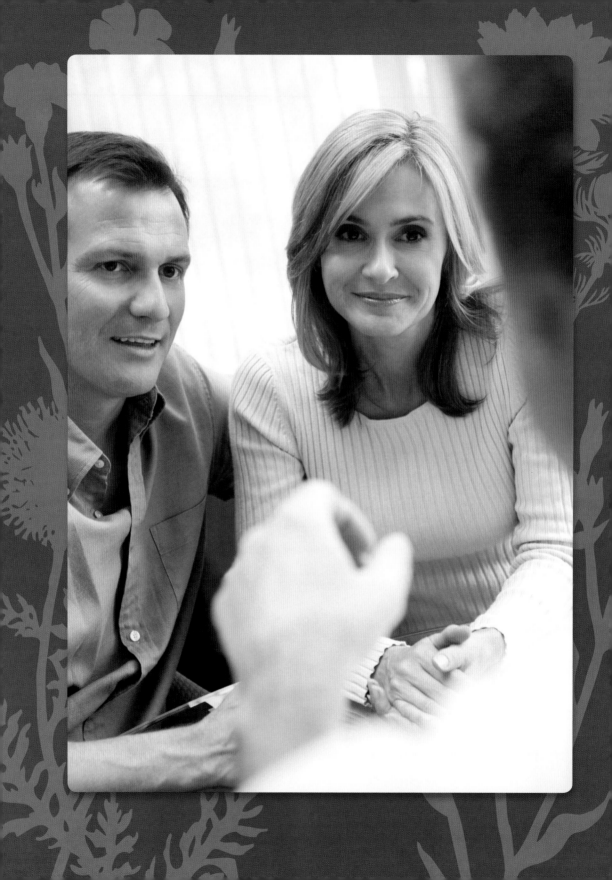

Control Point 20

Important Questions for Your Treatment Team

Control Point #20

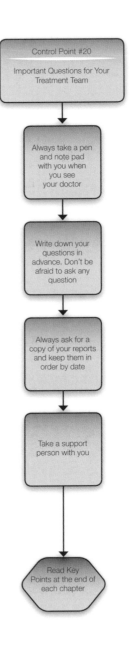

Control Point #20

Important Questions for Your
Treatment Team

Always take a pen
and note pad
with you when
you see
your doctor

Write down your
questions in
advance. Don't be
afraid to ask any
question

Always ask for a
copy of your reports
and keep them in
order by date

Take a support
person with you

Read Key
Points at the end of
each chapter

20

Important Questions for Your Treatment Team

Don't be afraid to ask questions. It is helpful to write your questions down before you see your treatment team. Listed below are some of the key questions that will help you get you started.

Before Your Surgery

- How sure are you that I have breast cancer?

- What is the stage of my cancer?

- Do I need any tests before surgery? (Common tests are mammogram, ultrasound, and fine needle and/or core biopsy)

- Do I need to have a mastectomy (breast removal)?

- Can I have a sentinel node biopsy?

- If have a sentinel node biopsy, how is it mapped and when and where is this done?

- If I have a sentinel node biopsy, will you do a quick test on it while I'm anesthetized to see if it's involved?

- Where do I go to check in for my procedure?

- How long do I fast before the surgery?

- Can any of my medications increase the risk of side effects from my surgery?

- Do you perform other types of surgery apart from breast surgery?

- If I have breast conservation, how will you place the scar?

- If I have a cancer that has only been found on the mammogram and can't be felt, how do you remove it? (A localization procedure is usually required using a mammogram or ultrasound to insert a guide wire or other marker to the cancer.)

- Can I see an oncologist before my surgery?

- Who is in your treatment team?

- Will doctors who specialize in breast cancer treat me?

- If I have a mastectomy, can I have an immediate reconstruction? If not, why not?

- Are there any clinical research trials or studies I should know about?

- How long will I be in the hospital?

- Will I have a drain inserted into my incision?

- Will I need to have stitches removed after the surgery?

- How long might it take me to recover from surgery?

- How much will surgery cost? (Check the costs of others services associated with surgery, such as the anesthetic or pathology testing, etc.)

- Will I have any pain with the treatment? What will be done about this?

- Is there a financial gap between what the government/insurance pays and your fee?

- Are there any side effects I should watch out for?

- When can I return to work?

- Are there any support groups who can help me?

After your surgery

- What type of breast cancer do I have? (The two most common types are invasive ductal or invasive lobular.)

- What is the grade of my cancer (1, 2, or 3)?

- What is the size of my cancer? (Check that only the invasive component is measured.)

- Is there an extensive intraductal component? (If yes, check that your margins are clear, and if they are, don't worry about this factor.)

- Are my margins clear?

- If yes, where is the closest margin, and how close in millimeters is the cancer to that margin?

- Is my tumor estrogen receptor-positive?

- What is the HER2 status of my tumor?

- Was my sentinel node involved?

- Have the final tests (immuno-histochemistry) come back on the sentinel node yet?

- If the sentinel node is involved,

how involved is it (isolated tumor cells, micro-metastasis, or a larger macro-metastasis)?

- How many nodes were dissected from my armpit?

- What was the total number of positive (or involved) nodes in my armpit?

- Do I need any further surgery?

- Do I need any further tests (such as a bone scan or a CT scan)?

- When will I see an oncologist? Or do I need to see an oncologist? If not, why not?

- Do I need physical therapy (physiotherapy) for my shoulder?

- When does my drain come out?

- How do I take care of my arm?

- When can I start to drive?

- When can I go back to work?

- I would like to have a second opinion. Can you refer me to someone else?

- Are there any support groups who can help me?

About your radiation therapy

- Do I need radiation therapy?

- Which areas of my body will get radiation therapy?

- How long is the course of the radiation therapy?

- Will I have to miss work?

- What times is the radiation therapy department open?

- How long does the radiation therapy planning session take to complete?

- What should I bring with me to the radiation therapy planning session? (Usually X-rays and maybe a consent form.)

- Is there any way to get help with traveling to and from the radiation therapy department?

- Where do I park when I'm having radiation therapy?

- Is there a fee for parking during radiation therapy?

- How long is the wait before radiation starts after my radiation therapy planning session?

- How many radiation therapy treatments will be given (usually 25–30)?

- What are the common side effects after radiation therapy?

- What are the uncommon side effects after radiation therapy?

- What are the long-term side effects after radiation therapy?

- Who will talk to me about looking after my skin and avoiding these side effects?

- How often will I be checked by you or your nurse or therapist while I'm having radiation therapy?

- Is there a number I can call if I'm worried about anything during my radiation therapy?

- Will the radiation therapy touch my heart?

- Should I give up smoking or drinking during my radiation therapy? (It's normally a good idea to give up smoking.)

- If I have radiation therapy to my chest wall, will this affect my chances of having a breast implant (reconstruction) later?

- When is the radiation therapy given in relation to chemotherapy?

- If I need chemotherapy after the radiation therapy, when should that start?

- How long does each radiation treatment take while I'm under the machine? (Usually, the radiation is turned on for about 50 seconds in each treatment location.)

- How long will I be in the radiation therapy department every day?

About hormonal treatments

- How do you decide which hormonal treatment is best for me?

- What side effects might I have during and after my treatment?

- What are the benefits of hormonal treatment for me?

- For how long should I take the hormonal treatment?

- Are there any other drugs I can have instead of tamoxifen?

- Do any of my other medications interfere with tamoxifen?

- What time of day do I take my hormonal treatment?

- Will tamoxifen stop my periods?

- Is tamoxifen enough for contraception?

- I've taken tamoxifen for five years; should I stop the drug or go onto an aromatase inhibitor?

- I've read about the new hormone therapies called aromatase inhibitors. Should I have these instead?

- If I use aromatase inhibitors, will you check my bone density?

- What are the main side effects of aromatase inhibitors?

- Will you check my blood vitamin D levels?

About chemotherapy

- What is the benefit of chemotherapy?

- What are my chances of survival if I have hormonal treatment instead?

- What drugs will I have? What "generation" of chemotherapy is it?

- How long will my course of treatment last?

- How often is the chemotherapy given (e.g. weekly, or once every two or three weeks)?

- How will I feel during my course of chemotherapy?

- What are the main side effects of chemotherapy?

- Are there any long-term side effects?

- How can I reduce the side effects?

- Will the treatment cause hair loss, and if so, will I lose hair all over my body?

- What can I do to help myself feel better during chemotherapy?

- Should I have a port?

- Will I go through menopause?

- What are my chances of infertility?

- Can fertility drugs affect my breast cancer?

- How much does IVF before chemotherapy cost?

- What's the chance of and how will I know if I get an infection?

- What do I do if I suspect an infection?

- When can I go back to work?

- Are there any support groups who can help me?

About Herceptin

- What is the benefit of Herceptin?

- What are my chances of survival if I use Herceptin?

- What drugs will I have with Herceptin?

- How long will my Herceptin course take?

- How often is the Herceptin given (e.g. weekly, or once every three weeks)?

- How will I feel during my course of Herceptin?

- What are the main side effects of Herceptin?

- How can I reduce the side effects?

- Are there any long-term side effects?

- What are the chances of heart damage with Herceptin?

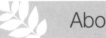

About follow-up

- How often do I need to come back for a follow-up check?

- Who should I see for my follow-up visits?

- What should I look out for?

- What tests do I need after my treatment?

- Who should I contact if I'm worried between my checks?

- How do I look after my arm?

- What do I do about contraception?

- Are there any support groups that can help me?

- When can I have a baby?

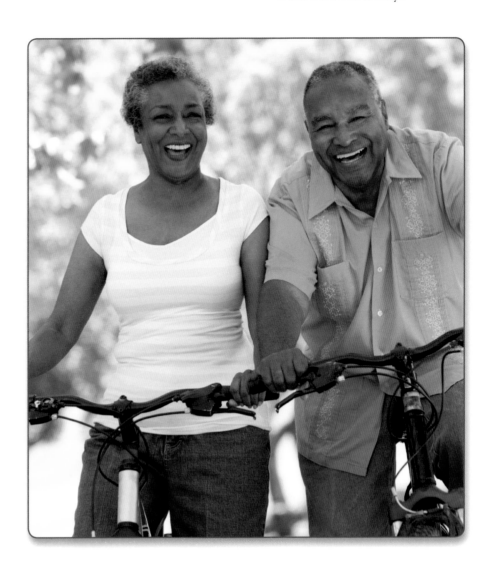

Now that Treatment is Over

Completing treatment is exciting but can also be stressful, particularly when the "umbilical cord" that had regularly linked you with your treatment team is suddenly cut. Having no more regular appointments sometimes increases fear and uncertainty.

It's only natural to feel this way, but it does get better with time. Life after breast cancer is going to be the topic of one of my next books. There's so much to cover that it will be a whole book on its own. In that book, I'll be talking about the role of genetics, tests, follow-up programs, contraception, pregnancy, sexuality, lymphedema, recurrence, staying positive, and the importance of nutrition and exercise.

For now, it's important to go to all of your scheduled follow-up appointments after treatment, and if you're worried, don't hesitate to make an earlier appointment. It can be scary at first, so keep in touch with your treatment team and your general practitioner. Try to coordinate your visits so that you see a different member of your team every four to six months, rather than seeing more than one member of your team within a few weeks.

The frequency of follow-up visits varies from treatment center to treatment center. Most problems tend to occur in the first five years, so the frequency of check-ups can be reduced to once per year after five years. You still need to have annual breast X-rays, and these may be followed up by an appointment with your family doctor.

Important aspects of follow-up include the following:

- Your doctor should ask you if you have any symptoms from the disease or its treatment

- Your doctor should rerview a mammogram with or without an ultrasound at every anniversary of your treatment

- You or your doctor may ask about any side effects of chemotherapy or hormonal treatment

- Have a physical exam to look for any lymphedema or recurrence. Your doctor will check under your armpits and above and below your collarbone area, your breast and chest wall area, and possibly other parts of your body such as your abdomen

- Organize an annual mammogram and/or breast ultrasound of one (if you've had a mastectomy) or both sides (if you've had breast conservation)

- Organize blood tests such as calcium and vitamin D levels and a bone density test, particularly if you are taking an aromatase inhibitor

- Have a yearly pelvic exam if you're taking tamoxifen, because this drug can very slightly increase your risk of uterine cancer. Be sure to tell your doctor right away about any abnormal vaginal bleeding you may have.

- Know that other tests, such as scans, are not required unless you have a specific new problem. Regular blood "tumor markers" are unreliable and generally not recommended

- Remember that most aches and pains are not cancer. You will get the odd back or muscle pain after gardening or exercise or just sitting at your desk for a long time. Don't be afraid to take some Tylenol/Panadol and see if the pain goes away. If a new pain is persistent, make an earlier appointment for a check-up. Most of the time, pain will not be related to your cancer, but if you don't feel right, see your doctor. If a pain, lump, or other symptom persists and won't go away, see your doctor.

- Maintain your emotional and physical wellbeing. Look after your diet, keep exercising, and try not to put on too much weight.

Don't forget that you need to stay in touch with your family doctor for routine checks that have nothing to do with breast cancer, such as blood pressure, Pap, and cholesterol checks. Talk to your doctor about the flu vaccine. After breast cancer, you can have the deactivated form of the vaccine, which is given as an injection into your muscle. Avoid the nasal spray flu vaccine, which contains weakened live flu viruses.

Please try to get back to as much of your normal life and routine as possible. I know that's easier said than done, but there are some simple things you can do. Plan weekends away, dates with your partner, and vacations with your family, and put off your doctors' appointments by a few weeks if they don't fit in with your vacation plans!

I really wish you all the very best and hope that *Breast Cancer: Taking Control* has helped you. Remember to enjoy some of life's pleasures—reading, gardening, eating and drinking well, walking, music, traveling, loving, community, family, and friends. Life goes on after breast cancer.

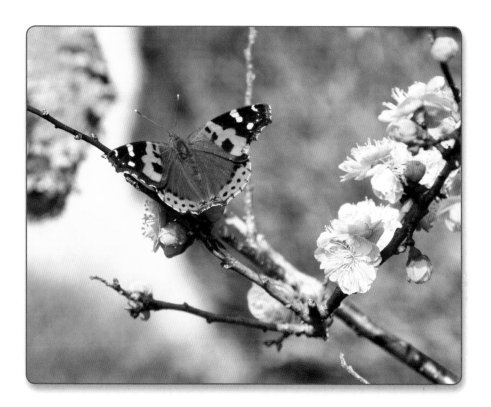

CONTROL POINT #20 – IMPORTANT QUESTIONS FOR YOUR TREATMENT TEAM

WARNING It can sometimes be both exciting and stressful after you finish your treatment and the "umbilical cord" with your treatment team is suddenly cut.

TIP Most aches and pains after your treatment are not breast cancer. Always ask for the name and contact number of the best person to call if you are worried.

REMEMBER There is no such thing as a silly question. If you're worried about anything at all, bring it to the attention of your doctor or nurse.

References

Arias, E. 2006. United States life tables, 2003. National Vital Statistics Reports 54: 1–40.

Axelsson, C.K. et al. 2009. Impact on regional recurrence and survival of axillary surgery in women with node-negative primary breast cancer. British Journal of Surgery 96: 40–46.

Baselga, J. et al. 2009. Phase II genomics study of ixabepilone as neoadjuvant treatment for breast cancer. Journal of Clinical Oncology 27: 526–534.

Bendz, I. and M. Fagevik Olsén. 2002. Evaluation of immediate versus delayed shoulder exercises after breast cancer surgery including lymph node dissection—a randomised controlled trial. Breast 11: 241–248.

Berger, J.C. et al. 2008. Pierre Robin sequence associated with first trimester fetal tamoxifen exposure. American Journal of Medical Genetics Part A 146A: 2141–2144.

Bohlius, J. et al. 2006. Recombinant human erythropoietins and cancer patients: updated meta-analysis of 57 studies including 9353 patients. Journal of the National Cancer Institute 98: 708–714.

Boyages, J. et al. 1990. Early breast cancer: predictors of breast recurrence for patients treated with conservative surgery and radiation therapy. Radiotherapy and Oncology 19: 29–41.

Boyages, J. and A. Langlands. 1998. Post-mastectomy radiation therapy: better late than never. Australian and New Zealand Journal of Surgery 68: 550–553.

Breast Cancer Action Group NSW. Breast Cancer Directory. http://www.bcagnsw.org.au/directory.htm (accessed March 1, 2009).

Buzdar, A..U. et al. 2005. Significantly higher pathologic complete remission rate after neoadjuvant therapy with trastuzumab, paclitaxel, and epirubicin chemotherapy: results of a randomized trial in human epidermal growth factor receptor 2-positive operable breast cancer. Journal of Clinical Oncology 23: 3676–3685.

Candace, R. and Darby, S.C. 2009. Cardiac disease and second lung cancer after radiotherapy for breast cancer. European Journal of Cancer 45: 420-421.

Chien, A.J. and P.E. Goss. 2006. Aromatase inhibitors and bone health in women with breast cancer. Journal of Clinical Oncology 24: 5305–5312.

Coombs, N. et al. 2007. A decision tool for predicting sentinel node accuracy from breast tumor size and grade. Breast Journal 13: 593–598.

Cserni, G. et al. 2003. European Working Group for Breast Screening Pathology. Pathological work-up of sentinel lymph nodes in breast cancer. Review of current data to be considered for the formulation of guidelines. European Journal of Cancer 39: 1654–1667.

Durrieu, G. et al. 2004. Fertility and outcomes of pregnancy after chemotherapy in a sample of childbearing aged women. Fundamental & Clinical Pharmacology 18: 573–579.

Early Breast Cancer Trialists' Collaborative Group (EBCTCG), 2005. Effects of radiotherapy and of differences in the extent of surgery for early breast cancer on local recurrence and 15-year survival: an overview of the randomised trials. Lancet 366: 2087–2106.

Ferraldeschi, R. and Newman, W.G. 2010. The impact of CYP2D6 genotyping on tamoxifen treatment Pharmaceuticals 3: 1122–1138.

Felson, D.T. and S.R. Cummings. 2005. Aromatase inhibitors and the syndrome of arthralgias with estrogen deprivation. Arthritis and Rheumatism 52: 2594–2598.

Fisher, B. et al. 2002. Twenty-year follow-up of a randomized trial comparing total mastectomy, lumpectomy, and lumpectomy plus irradiation for the treatment of invasive breast cancer. New England Journal of Medicine 347: 1233–1241.

Galea, M.H. et al. 1992. The Nottingham Prognostic Index in primary breast cancer. Breast Cancer Research and Treatment 22: 207–219.

Geyer, C.E. et al. 2006. Lapatinib plus capecitabine for HER2-positive advanced breast cancer. New England Journal of Medicine 355: 2733–2743.

Gnant, M. et al. 2008. Adjuvant endocrine therapy plus zoledronic acid in premenopausal women with early-stage breast cancer: 5-year follow-up of the ABCSG-12 bone-mineral density substudy. Lancet Oncology 9: 840–849.

Gnant, M. et al. 2009. Endocrine therapy plus zoledronic acid in premenopausal breast cancer. New England Journal of Medicine 360: 679–691.

Goldhirsch, A. et al. 2009. Thresholds for therapies: highlights of the St Gallen International Expert Consensus on the primary therapy of early breast cancer 2009. Annals of Oncology 20: 1319–1329.

Goodwin, P.J. et al. 1999. Risk of menopause during the first year after breast cancer diagnosis. Journal of Clinical Oncology 17: 2365–2370.

Goodwin, P.J. et al. 2008 Annual Meeting Proceedings, American Society of Clinical Oncology. Frequency of vitamin D deficiency at breast cancer diagnosis and association with risk of distant recurrence and death in a prospective cohort study of T1-3, N0-1, M0 B. Journal of Clinical Oncology, 2008 ASCO Annual Meeting Proceedings, 26 (May 20 suppl); abstr 511.

Goss, P.E. et al. 2005. Randomized trial of letrozole following tamoxifen as extended adjuvant therapy in receptor-positive breast cancer: updated findings from NCIC CTG MA.17. Journal of the National Cancer Institute 97: 1262–1271.

Gradishar, W. et al. 2000. Effects of high dose raloxifene in selected patients with advanced breast carcinoma. Cancer 88: 2047–2053.

Halyard, M.Y. et al. 2006. Adjuvant radiotherapy (RT) and trastuzumab in stage I-IIA breast cancer: Toxicity data from North Central Cancer Treatment Group Phase III trial N9831. Journal of Clinical Oncology, ASCO Annual Meeting Proceedings Part I. Vol. 24 (18S): abstr 523.

Heaney, R.P. et. al. 2000. Bioavailability of the calcium in fortified soy imitation milk, with some observations on method. American Journal of Clinical Nutrition 71: 1166–1169.

Hickey, M. et al. 2009. Breast cancer in young women and its impact on reproductive function. Human Reproduction Update 15: 323–339.

Hudis, C. 2002. Breast cancer and leukemia: the forest for the trees? Annals of Surgical Oncology 9: 717–718.

Jenkins, V. et al. 2008. Effects of anastrozole on cognitive performance in postmenopausal women: a randomised, double-blind chemoprevention trial (IBIS II). Lancet Oncology 9: 953–961.

Joensuu, H. et al. 2006. Adjuvant docetaxel or vinorelbine with or without trastuzumab for breast cancer. New England Journal of Medicine 354: 809–820.

Kendall, A. et al. 2006. Caution: vaginal estradiol appears to be contraindicated in postmenopausal women on adjuvant aromatase inhibitors. Annals of Oncology 17: 584–587.

Kenemans, P. et al. 2009. Safety and efficacy of tibolone in breast-cancer patients with vasomotor symptoms: a double-blind, randomised, non-inferiority trial. Lancet Oncology 10: 135–146.

Kennedy, S.H. et al. 2000. Antidepressant-induced sexual dysfunction during treatment with moclobemide, paroxetine, sertraline, and venlafaxine. Journal of Clinical Psychiatry 61: 276–281.

King, M.T. et al. 2000. Quality of life three months and one year after first treatment for early stage breast cancer: Influence of treatment and patient characteristics. Quality of Life Research 9: 789–800.

Kroman, N. et al. 1997. Should women be advised against pregnancy after breast-cancer treatment? Lancet 350: 319–322.

Krychman, M. 2009. 100 questions & answers about women's sexual wellness and vitality: A practical guide for the woman seeking sexual fulfillment. Boston: Jones and Bartlett.

Lee, S.J. et al. 2006. American Society of Clinical Oncology recommendations on fertility preservation in cancer patients. Journal of Clinical Oncology 24: 2917–2931.

Leong, C. et al. 2004. Effect of margins on ipsilateral breast tumor recurrence after breast conservation therapy for lymph node-negative breast carcinoma. Cancer 100: 1823–1832.

Mansel, R.E. et al. 2009: Detection of breast cancer metastasis in sentinel lymph nodes using intra-operative real time GeneSearch BLN Assay in the operating room: results of the Cardiff study. Breast Cancer Research and Treatment 115: 595–600.

Marchal, C, et al. 1999: Nine breast angiosarcomas after conservative treatment for breast carcinoma: a survey from French Comprehensive Cancer Centers, International Journal of Radiation Oncology Biolgy Physics 44: 113-119

Matsumoto, M. 2006. Inhibition of paclitaxel-induced A-fiber hypersensitization by gabapentin. Journal of Pharmacological Experimental Therapeutics 318: 735–740.

McMahon, B. and J. Worcester. 1966: Age at menopause. United States 1960–1962. Vital and Health Statistics Series 11: 1–20.

Morris, J. and G.T. Royle. 1987. Choice of surgery for early breast cancer: pre- and postoperative levels of clinical anxiety and depression in patients and their husbands. British Journal of Surgery 74: 1017–1019.

Mourits, M.J.E. et al. 2007. Beware of amenorrhea during tamoxifen: it may be a wolf in sheep's clothing. Journal of Clinical Oncology 25: 3787–3788.

Murray, N. and R.J. Klasa. 2008. Reconsideration of American Society of Clinical Oncology/American Society of Hematology Erythropoiesis-stimulating agent guidelines. Journal of Clinical Oncology 26: 3096–3097.

National Cancer Institute. 2003. http://www.cancer.gov/cancertopics/eatinghints (accessed 1 March 2009).

National Cancer Institute. 2009. http://cancercenters.cancer.gov/cancer_centers/cancer-centers-names.html (accessed 29 May 2009).

NSW Cancer Council November. 2008. http://www.cancercouncil.com.au/html/prevention/sunsmart/downloads/Vitamin%20D%20.indd.pdf (accessed 26 May 2009).

Nutrition Coordinating Center. Nutrition Data System for Research, Version 4.06/34. Minneapolis: University of Minnesota, 2003.

Pae CU. et al. 2005. Paroxetine-associated spontaneous sexual stimulation. International Clinical Psychopharmacology 20: 339–341.

Park, C.C. et al. 2000. Outcome at 8 years after breast-conserving surgery and radiation therapy for invasive breast cancer: influence of margin status and systemic therapy on local recurrence. Journal of Clinical Oncology 18: 1668–1675.

Patani, N. and Mokbel K. 2008. Oncological and aesthetic considerations of skin-sparing mastectomy. Breast Cancer Research and Treatment 111:391–403.

Pennington, J., A. Bowes and H. Church. Bowes & Church's Food Values of Portions Commonly Used, 17th ed. Philadelphia: Lippincott Williams & Wilkins, 1998.

Pennington, J.A. and J.S. Douglass. Bowes and Church's Food Values of Portions Commonly Used, 18th ed. Philadelphia: Lippincott Williams & Wilkins, 2004.

Petrek, J.A. et al. 2006. Incidence, time course, and determinants of menstrual bleeding after breast cancer treatment: a prospective study. Journal of Clinical Oncology 24: 1045–1051.

Poortmans, P.M. et al. 2008. The addition of a boost dose on the primary tumour bed after lumpectomy in breast conserving treatment for breast cancer. A summary of the results of EORTC 22881-10882 'boost versus no boost' trial, Cancer/Radiotherapie 12: 565-570.

Recht, A. 2009. Contralateral prophylactic mastectomy: caveat emptor. Journal of Clinical Oncology 27: 1347–1349.

Robert, N.J. and W. Eiermann et al. 2007. BCIRG 006: Docetaxel and trastuzumab-based regimens improve DFS and OS over AC-T in node positive and high risk node negative HER2 positive early breast cancer patients: Quality of life (QOL) at 36 months follow-up. Journal of Clinical Oncology, ASCO Annual Meeting Proceedings 25; 18S: 19647.

Romond, E.H. et al. 2005. Trastuzumab plus adjuvant chemotherapy for operable HER2-positive breast cancer. New England Journal of Medicine 353: 1673–1684.

Schwartz, G. et al. 2006. Consensus conference on breast conservation. Journal of the American College of Surgeons 203: 198–207.

Smith I, et al. 2006. Adjuvant aromatase inhibitors for early breast cancer after chemotherapy-induced amenorrhoea: caution and suggested guidelines. Journal of Clinical Oncology 24: 2444–2447.

US Department of Agriculture, Agricultural Research Service. USDA Nutrient Database for Standard Reference, Release 16, 2003. http://www.ars.usda.gov/research/publications/publications.htm?seq_no_115=151898 (accessed 1 March 2009).

Visvanathan, K. et al. 2009. ASCO clinical practice guideline update on the use of pharmacologic interventions including tamoxifen, raloxifene, and aromatase inhibition for breast cancer risk reduction. Journal of Clinical Oncology 27: 3235–3258.

Vahtsevanos, K. et al. 2009. Longitudinal cohort study of risk factors in cancer patients of bisphosphonate-related osteonecrosis of the jaw. Journal of Clinical Oncology 27:5356-5362.

Whelan, T.J. et al. 2010. Long-term results of hypofractionated radiation therapy for breast cancer. New England Journal of Medicine 362: 513-520.

Credits

Cover and book design: Mishu Rahman (Shahanawaz A. Rahman): mishu@eyesometric.com

Editing: Rachel Haimowitz:metarachel@gmail.com

Production proofing: Olivia Wroth: olivia@superscriptwriting.com.au

Indexing consultancy: Glenda Browne: glendabrowne@optusnet.com.au

Figures 4, 22, 33–36, 38, 39–42, 55 (right), 63–65, 81, 82, 84–86, 90–94, © BoyCare Pty Ltd./Mishu Rahman

Figures 5, 6 and 43 © BoyCare Pty Ltd./Margaret Mapperson: mjmartistry@gmail.com

Figures 9–12, 22–25, 29–31, 45, 46, 53, 56–62, 68, 70, 71, 76–79 and Photo page 364 (Kastellorizo, my father's birth place), © BoyCare Pty Ltd. All clinical photos have model release forms assigned to BoyCare Pty Ltd.

Figure of cherry blossom, page 79 and camelia, page 229, from Matsuyama, Shikoku, Japan compliments of Fiona Collison. Figure of butterfly, page 327, from Tsumago–juku, Japan compliments of Lachlan Grant.

Shutterstock Images, under license: Figures 2 (Mati Dovner), 69 and CP#11 (Image ID: 10766794), 17 (Michael Spivak), 20 (ID: 2485991), 32 (Preobrazhenski), 35 (Darren Baker), 66, Photo page 324, CP#20 (Monkey Business Image), 80(Annette Shaff), Photograph page 22 (Bochkarev Photography), CP#2 (Elena Elisseeva), CP#4 (Marin), CP#6 (Loskutnikov), CP#8 (Jose AS Reyes), CP#9 (Greg Epperson), CP#16 (Kiselev Andrey Valerevich), CP#18(Timurpix), CP#19(Andi Berger), Photos: page 36 (top) (Moiseeva Galina Gavrilovna), page 36–bottom (Yellowj), page 131 (Cisco Freeze), page155 (Yuri Arcurs).

iStockphoto, under license:Cover Page and CP#3: (Chris Gramly), "Mel's story"(Kristian sekulic), CP#1 (Sean Locke), CP#7 and photo page 144 (Diane Diederich), CP #10 (Jacob Wackerhausen), CP#12(P.Rao), CP#13 (olly), CP#14 (Mark Kostich), CP#15 (absolut_100), Figures:1 (Lars Christensen), 3 (Chistoprudov Dmitriy Gennadievich), 7 (Sternstunden), 8 (Darren Baker), 16 (Joseph Jean Rolland Dubé), 18(Debi Bishop), 19 (Mark Weiss), 21 and 26–28(JazzIRT modified by Mishu Rahman) 67(Dave White), 83 (John Woodworth), 88 (Dawn Poland), 89(Gulcan Yasemin Sumer), photo page 195 (forestpath) Figure 2 is also by permission of Seven Towns Ltd.

Figure 44 compliments A/Prof. Elizabeth Salisbury, Figure 74 and photo page 253, with permission Sydney West Area Health Service

Figure 47, 49, 51 BARBIE ® Registered Trademark of Mattel Inc. El Segundo, California U.S.A and ® Registered Trademark of Nearly Me Technologies, Inc. ©2009 NMT.All Rights Reserved. With permission: Nearly Me Technologies, Inc., Waco, Texas, U.S.A.

Figure 75 with permission of Sydney Radiotherapy and Oncology Centre
Figure 37 with permission of GE Healthcare © General Electric Company 2009
Figures 48, 50, 52, and 54 (and CP#5) compliments of Amoena Australia Pty Ltd.
Figure 55 (left) reproduced with permission from Allergan © Allergan 2009
Figure 72 and table 16 with permission of and personal communication with Dr. Peter Ravdin
Figure 73 Image courtesy of Varian Medical Systems of Palo Alto, California. © 2009, Varian Medical Systems. All rights reserved.
Figure 87 and CP#17, © Simon Jarratt/Corbis
Figures 90–93 and table 3 reprinted with permission from the American Society of Clinical Oncology
Figure 95–96 courtesy of Dragons Abreast Central Coast and Australia respectively

Appendix #1 Dragons Abreast

I'd like to give a plug to the fabulous work that organizations like Dragon Abreast do to help people cope both emotionally and physically. Go to their main web site:

www.abreastinaboat.com/, or www.dragonsabreast.com.au/ in Australia.

Dr. Don McKenzie, a sports medicine physician at the University of British Columbia, launched "Abreast in a Boat" in 1996 to test the myth that repetitive upper-body exercise in women who were treated for breast cancer encourages lymphedema (swelling of the arm because of blocked lymphatics in the treated armpit).

Dr. McKenzie believed that by following a special exercise and training program, women could avoid lymphedema and enjoy active, full lives. Dr McKenzie's theory was proven correct. Among the women who participated in Abreast in a Boat, no new cases of lymphedema occurred and none of the existing cases became worse. There is now a worldwide movement of breast cancer survivors paddling dragon boats, known in Australia as "Dragons Abreast," and by various names in the US See www.abreastinaboat.com/HTML/contacts.htm#us for various clubs in the US.

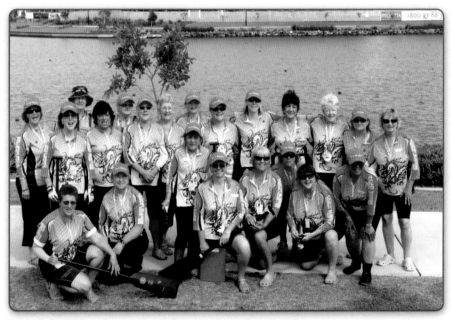

Figure 95: Central Coast Dragons Abreast Crew, New South Wales, Australia.

Dragons Abreast teams are comprised of breast cancer survivors of various ages and a great variety of backgrounds, athletic abilities, and interests. They are founded on the principles of participation and inclusiveness, and not competitive outcome (Figures 95 and 96).

Dragons Abreast members provide a "face" for the breast cancer statistics while spreading the message of breast cancer awareness through participation in the wonderful and strenuous sport of dragon boat racing. High on their list of priorities is having fun, trying new things, meeting interesting people, and being involved in a challenging physical activity while promoting breast cancer awareness. Give it a go.

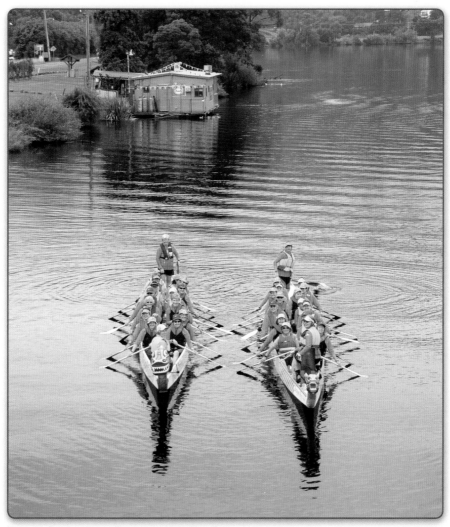

Figure 96: Dragons Abreast Team on the Huon River, Tasmania, Australia.

Appendix #2 Other Women with Breast Cancer

Name	Walk of Life
Christina Applegate	American actress
Shirley Temple Black	Oscar-winning American child star and former US ambassador
Raelene Boyle	Australian athlete
Bette Davis	American Oscar-winning actress
Belinda Emmett	Australian actress
Betty Ford	Former US First Lady
Ruth Mosko Handler	American creator of BARBIE® Doll and NEARLY ME® mastectomy products
Linda McCartney	American singer, activist, and wife of former British Beatles member Sir Paul McCartney
Jane Louise McGrath (née Steele)	British-born Australian cancer support campaigner, and the wife of Australian cricket fast bowler Glenn McGrath.
Kylie Minogue	Australian singer and actress
Olivia Newton-John	U.K./Australian singer and actress
Sandra Day O'Connor	Former US Supreme Court justice
Nancy Reagan	Former US First Lady
Lynn Redgrave	Oscar nominated British–American actress
Richard Roundtree	American actor and breast cancer advocate
Carly Simon	American singer

Appendix #3 Useful Websites

Organisation	Website
American Cancer Society	www.cancer.org
American Society of Clinical Oncology	www.plwc.org
Amoena—for breast styles and prostheses	www.amoena.org
American Society for Therapeutic Radiology and Oncology Patient Site	www.rtanswers.org
Breastcancer.org	www.breastcancer.org
Breast Cancer Action Group NSW	www.bcagnsw.org.au/

Appendix #3 Useful Websites

Organisation	Website
Breast Cancer Care (U.K.)	www.breastcancercare.org.uk
Breast Cancer Network of Strength (formerly Y-ME)	www.networkofstrength.org
Breast Cancer Network Australia	www.bcna.org.au
Cancerbackup (U.K.)	www.cancerbackup.org.uk
Cancer Care	www.cancercare.org
Cancer Hope Network	www.cancerhopenetwork.org
Cancer Research UK	www.cancerhelp.org.uk
Clinical Trials (USA)	www.clinicaltrials.gov
ENCORE Gentle Exercise Program	www.ywca.org or www.ywcaencore.org.au
Fertile Hope—Network for cancer patients	www.fertilehope.org
Living Beyond Breast Cancer	www.lbbc.org
Look Good Feel Better	www.lookgoodfeelbetter.org
My parent's cancer	www.myparentscancer.com.au/home.html
National Alliance of Breast Cancer Organization (NABCO)	www.nabco.org
National Breast and Ovarian Cancer Centre (Australia)	www.nbocc.org.au
National Breast Cancer Coalition	www.stopbreastcancer.org
National Cancer Institute	www.cancer.gov/cancertopics/types/breast
National Comprehensive Cancer Network	www.nccn.org
National Lymphedema Network	www.lymphnet.org
NEARLY ME® mastectomy products	www.nearlyme.org
Office of Cancer Complementary and Alternative Medicine	www.cancer.gov/cam/health_patients.html
Oncolink	www.oncolink.org
Patient Advocate Foundation	www.patientadvocate.org
People Living with Cancer	www.peoplelivingwithcancer.org
Quackwatch—Health-related frauds and myths	www.quackwatch.org
Resolve: The National Infertility Association	www.resolve.org
Radiological Society of North America (RSNA)	www.radiologyinfo.org
Susan G. Komen Breast Cancer Foundation	www.komen.org
Westmead Breast Cancer Institute (Australia)	www.bci.org.au
Women's Cancer Network	www.wcn.org

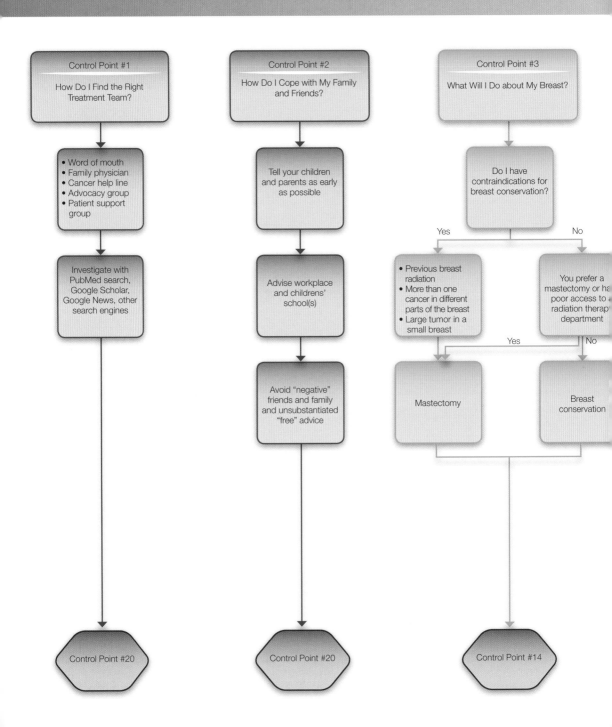

Control Point #1

How Do I Find the Right Treatment Team?

- Word of mouth
- Family physician
- Cancer help line
- Advocacy group
- Patient support group

Investigate with PubMed search, Google Scholar, Google News, other search engines

Control Point #20

Control Point #2

How Do I Cope with My Family and Friends?

Tell your children and parents as early as possible

Advise workplace and childrens' school(s)

Avoid "negative" friends and family and unsubstantiated "free" advice

Control Point #20

Control Point #3

What Will I Do about My Breast?

Do I have contraindications for breast conservation?

Yes — No

- Previous breast radiation
- More than one cancer in different parts of the breast
- Large tumor in a small breast

You prefer a mastectomy or ha poor access to radiation therapy department

Yes — No

Mastectomy

Breast conservation

Control Point #14

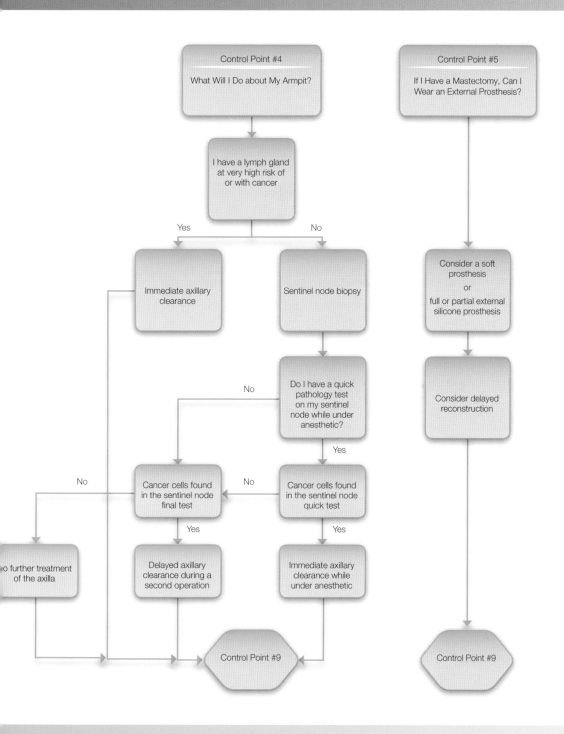

Control Point #4

What Will I Do about My Armpit?

I have a lymph gland at very high risk of or with cancer

Yes

No

Immediate axillary clearance

Sentinel node biopsy

Do I have a quick pathology test on my sentinel node while under anesthetic?

No

Yes

Cancer cells found in the sentinel node final test

No

Cancer cells found in the sentinel node quick test

No

Yes

Yes

No further treatment of the axilla

Delayed axillary clearance during a second operation

Immediate axillary clearance while under anesthetic

Control Point #9

Control Point #5

If I Have a Mastectomy, Can I Wear an External Prosthesis?

Consider a soft prosthesis

or

full or partial external silicone prosthesis

Consider delayed reconstruction

Control Point #9

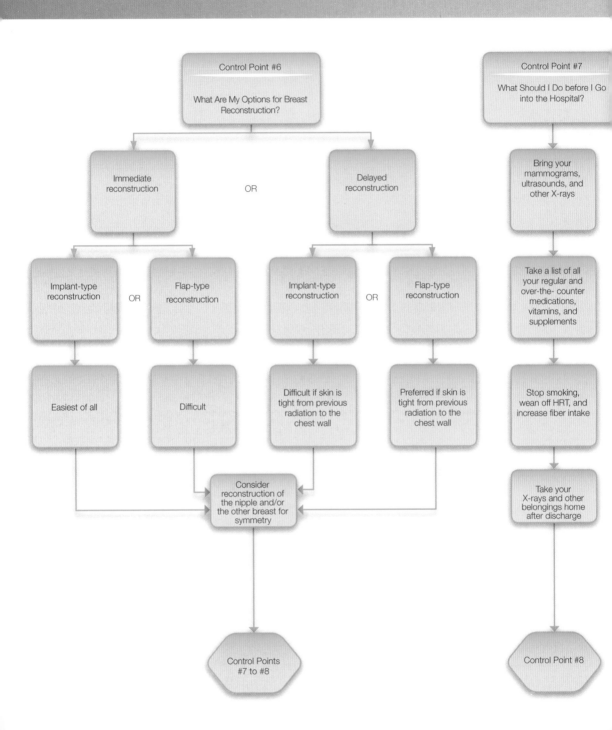

Control Point #6

What Are My Options for Breast Reconstruction?

Immediate reconstruction

OR

Delayed reconstruction

Implant-type reconstruction

OR

Flap-type reconstruction

Implant-type reconstruction

OR

Flap-type reconstruction

Easiest of all

Difficult

Difficult if skin is tight from previous radiation to the chest wall

Preferred if skin is tight from previous radiation to the chest wall

Consider reconstruction of the nipple and/or the other breast for symmetry

Control Points #7 to #8

Control Point #7

What Should I Do before I Go into the Hospital?

Bring your mammograms, ultrasounds, and other X-rays

Take a list of all your regular and over-the- counter medications, vitamins, and supplements

Stop smoking, wean off HRT, and increase fiber intake

Take your X-rays and other belongings home after discharge

Control Point #8

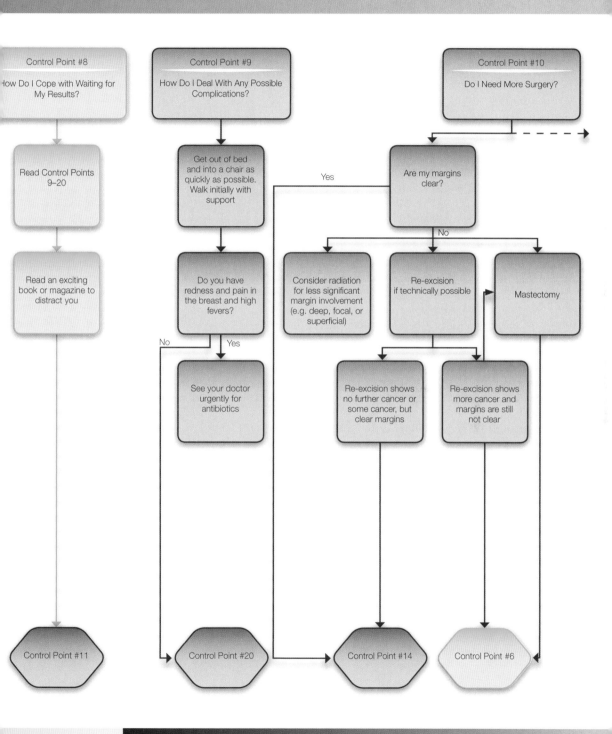

Control Point #8

How Do I Cope with Waiting for My Results?

↓

Read Control Points 9–20

↓

Read an exciting book or magazine to distract you

↓

Control Point #11

Control Point #9

How Do I Deal With Any Possible Complications?

↓

Get out of bed and into a chair as quickly as possible. Walk initially with support

↓

Do you have redness and pain in the breast and high fevers?

No / Yes

See your doctor urgently for antibiotics

↓

Control Point #20

Control Point #10

Do I Need More Surgery?

Are my margins clear?

Yes / No

Consider radiation for less significant margin involvement (e.g. deep, focal, or superficial)

Re-excision if technically possible

Mastectomy

Re-excision shows no further cancer or some cancer, but clear margins

Re-excision shows more cancer and margins are still not clear

↓

Control Point #14

Control Point #6

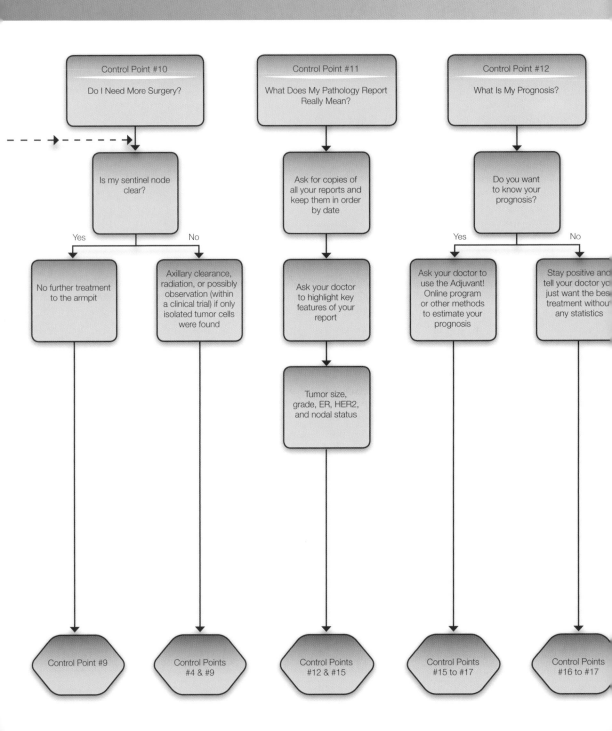

Control Point #10

Do I Need More Surgery?

Control Point #11

What Does My Pathology Report Really Mean?

Control Point #12

What Is My Prognosis?

Is my sentinel node clear?

Ask for copies of all your reports and keep them in order by date

Do you want to know your prognosis?

Yes | No

No further treatment to the armpit

Axillary clearance, radiation, or possibly observation (within a clinical trial) if only isolated tumor cells were found

Ask your doctor to highlight key features of your report

Yes | No

Ask your doctor to use the Adjuvant! Online program or other methods to estimate your prognosis

Stay positive and tell your doctor you just want the best treatment without any statistics

Tumor size, grade, ER, HER2, and nodal status

Control Point #9

Control Points #4 & #9

Control Points #12 & #15

Control Points #15 to #17

Control Points #16 to #17

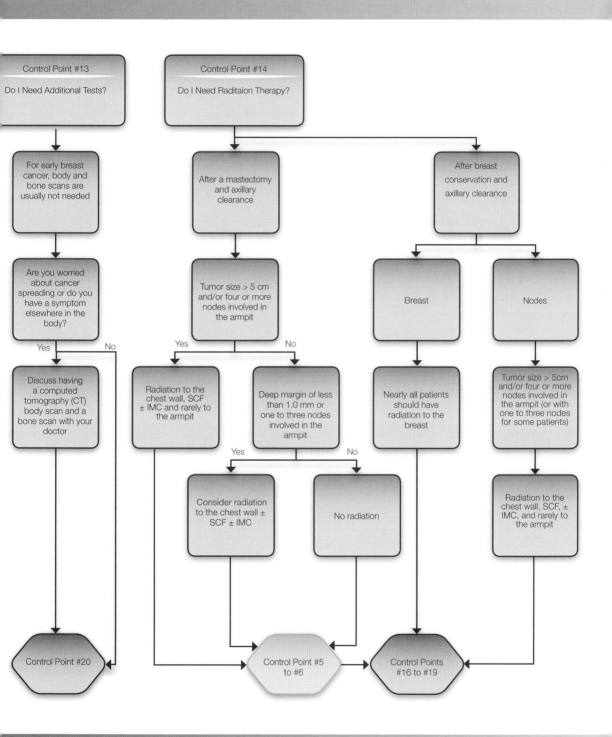

Control Point #13

Do I Need Additional Tests?

Control Point #14

Do I Need Raditaion Therapy?

For early breast cancer, body and bone scans are usually not needed

After a mastectomy and axillary clearance

After breast conservation and axillary clearance

Are you worried about cancer spreading or do you have a symptom elsewhere in the body?

Yes　No

Tumor size > 5 cm and/or four or more nodes involved in the armpit

Yes　No

Breast

Nodes

Discuss having a computed tomography (CT) body scan and a bone scan with your doctor

Radiation to the chest wall, SCF ± IMC and rarely to the armpit

Deep margin of less than 1.0 mm or one to three nodes involved in the armpit

Nearly all patients should have radiation to the breast

Tumor size > 5cm and/or four or more nodes involved in the armpit (or with one to three nodes for some patients)

Yes　No

Consider radiation to the chest wall ± SCF ± IMC

No radiation

Radiation to the chest wall, SCF, ± IMC, and rarely to the armpit

Control Point #20

Control Point #5 to #6

Control Points #16 to #19

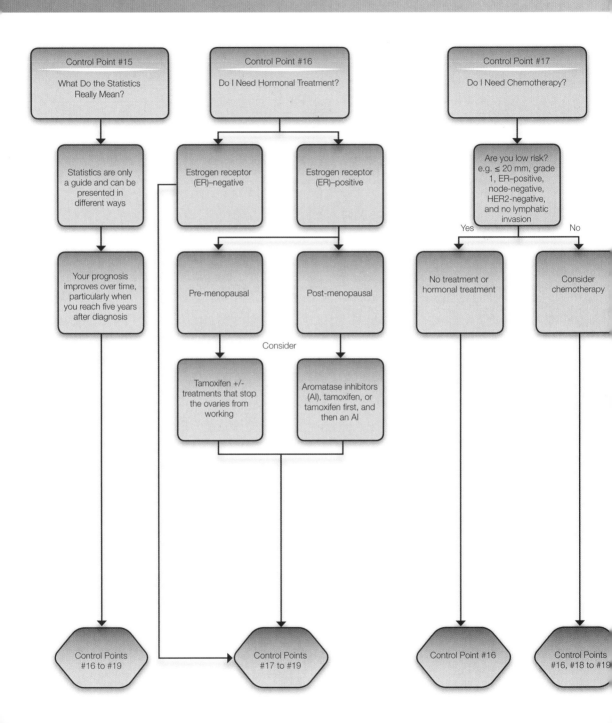

Control Point #15

What Do the Statistics Really Mean?

Statistics are only a guide and can be presented in different ways

Your prognosis improves over time, particularly when you reach five years after diagnosis

Control Points #16 to #19

Control Point #16

Do I Need Hormonal Treatment?

Estrogen receptor (ER)–negative

Estrogen receptor (ER)–positive

Pre-menopausal

Post-menopausal

Consider

Tamoxifen +/- treatments that stop the ovaries from working

Aromatase inhibitors (AI), tamoxifen, or tamoxifen first, and then an AI

Control Points #17 to #19

Control Point #17

Do I Need Chemotherapy?

Are you low risk? e.g. ≤ 20 mm, grade 1, ER–positive, node-negative, HER2-negative, and no lymphatic invasion

Yes   No

No treatment or hormonal treatment

Consider chemotherapy

Control Point #16

Control Points #16, #18 to #19

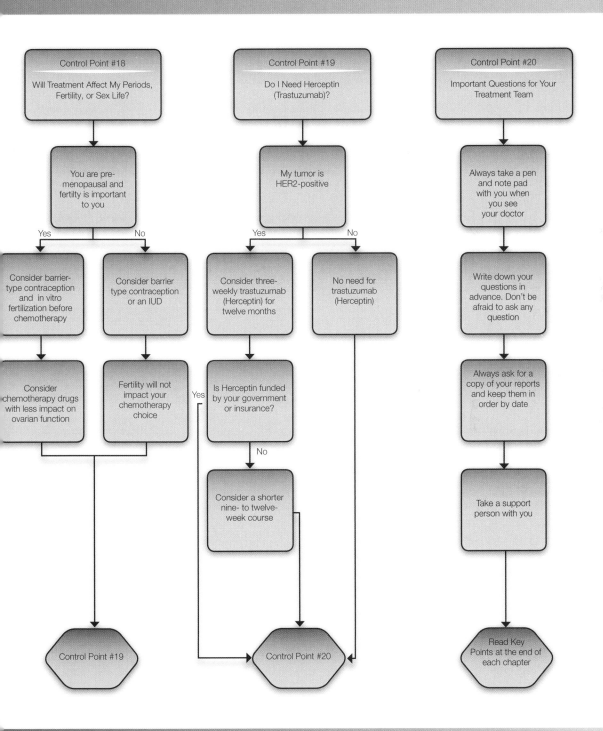

Control Point #18

Will Treatment Affect My Periods, Fertility, or Sex Life?

↓

You are pre-menopausal and fertilty is important to you

Yes / No

Consider barrier-type contraception and in vitro fertilization before chemotherapy

Consider barrier type contraception or an IUD

Consider chemotherapy drugs with less impact on ovarian function

Fertility will not impact your chemotherapy choice

Control Point #19

Control Point #19

Do I Need Herceptin (Trastuzumab)?

↓

My tumor is HER2-positive

Yes / No

Consider three-weekly trastuzumab (Herceptin) for twelve months

No need for trastuzumab (Herceptin)

Is Herceptin funded by your government or insurance?

Yes / No

Consider a shorter nine- to twelve-week course

Control Point #20

Control Point #20

Important Questions for Your Treatment Team

↓

Always take a pen and note pad with you when you see your doctor

Write down your questions in advance. Don't be afraid to ask any question

Always ask for a copy of your reports and keep them in order by date

Take a support person with you

Read Key Points at the end of each chapter

Glossary

ABSCESS: A boil or collection of pus caused by infection.

AC (doxorubicin and cyclophosphamide): A common type of chemotherapy regimen or recipe combining two different drugs; also known as Adriamycin and Cytoxan.

ADJUVANT: Additional treatment given after surgery to increase the chances of survival, including hormonal treatment, chemotherapy, or radiation therapy.

ALOPECIA: Loss of hair from the use of chemotherapy.

ANEMIA: The presence of a low number of red cells in the blood; it can cause tiredness.

AREOLA: The dark skin around your nipple.

AROMATASE: A special chemical in the body that produces estrogen after you have gone through menopause. Aromatase is part of a family of chemicals called enzymes.

AROMATASE INHIBITOR (AI): A drug that reduces the production of estrogen in the body after you have gone through menopause. Three drugs in this class are available: anastrozole (Arimidex), letrozole (Femara), and exemestane (Aromasin).

ATYPIA: A change in the lining of the ducts in your breast wherein they start to look "atypical" or abnormal.

AVASTIN: Avastin, or bevacizumab, is a monoclonal antibody for patients with advanced breast cancer. It works by blocking the formation of new blood vessels (angiogenesis) that feed the cancer.

AXILLA: The armpit.

AXILLARY CLEARANCE: Surgery that removes a fat pad from under your armpit that contains some or all of the lymph glands.

AXILLARY DISSECTION: SEE AXILLARY CLEARANCE

BIOPSY: A test involving the removal of cells (fine-needle biopsy) or tissue (core biopsy) for diagnosis.

BIOIMPEDANCE: A method of determining the presence of bodily fluids such as lymph by measuring how well your arm conducts a small electric current.

BISPHOSPHONATES: Drugs that work by reducing the activity of osteoclasts (cells that break down bone) and helping the osteoblasts (cells that build up bone). They are used when you have osteoporosis or breast cancer that has spread to the bone.

BLOOD COUNT: A blood test that measures the number of red and white cells and platelets just before or midway through a course of chemotherapy. These cells are usually at their lowest point two weeks after each course.

BONE MINERAL DENSITY: A measure of how strong your bones are, using a test that measures the amount of minerals contained in a certain volume of bone. Bone mineral density measurements are used to diagnose bone thinning or osteoporosis. (see "OSTEOPOROSIS")

BONE SCAN: A type of X-ray scan where a small trace of radioactivity is injected into a vein in your arm and is then taken up by all your bones. Cancer appears as a "hot spot" or abnormal area of intensity in the subsequent scan.

BOOST: An extra course of radiation to the tumor bed.

BRCA1 OR BRCA2 GENE: Human genes that belong to a class of genes known as tumor suppressors. Mutation or "defects" of these genes has been linked to hereditary breast and ovarian cancer.

BREAST CONSERVATION: SEE "LUMPECTOMY"

BREAST PROSTHESIS: An artificial breast or breast form, usually made of silicone gel, that can be worn inside your bra or inserted by a plastic surgeon permanently under your chest muscles (a breast implant) following a mastectomy.

CANDIDA: see "THRUSH"

CAPSULITIS: thickening that can occur around an internal breast prosthesis or implant, particularly if radiation is given.

CATARACT: Clouding of the lens inside the eye.

CELLULITIS: A rapid onset, spreading infection of the deep tissues of the skin and muscle. Cellulitis causes the skin to become very hot and tender and may also cause fever, chills, and swollen and tender lymph glands.

CHEMOTHERAPY (chemo, cytotoxic drugs, anti-cancer drugs): The use of drugs, usually given intravenously, to kill, slow, or stall the growth of cancer cells.

CHEMOTHERAPY BRAIN: Forgetfulness that can occur after chemotherapy.

CLAVICLE: The breastbone at the base of the neck.

CLINICAL TRIAL: Research, conducted with your permission, that usually involves a comparison of two or more treatments (an existing treatment is compared to a new and potentially better treatment). Which patients receive the old treatment and the new treatment is randomly allocated by a computer.

CMF (cyclophosphamide, methotrexate, and fluorouracil): A common type of chemotherapy regimen or recipe combining three different drugs; also known as Cytoxan, Mexate, and fluorouracil (5-FU or Adrucil).

COLLOID CARCINOMA: SEE "MUCINOUS CARCINOMAS"

CORDING: An uncommon side effect after surgery, appearing as a painful string-like tissue extending down the inner arm from the armpit to the hand. It is usually treated with vitamin E cream, massage, and physiotherapy.

CORE BIOPSY: The sampling of breast tissue with a needle larger than that used in a fine needle biopsy. A core biopsy produces a tiny cylinder or core of tissue for examination by a pathologist. It's like taking a core from an apple or the soil to work out whether a lump or abnormal mammogram could be cancer.

CT (COMPUTED TOMOGRAPHY) SCAN: An X-ray test taken from different angles of a part of the body. These images are combined by a computer to make cross-sectional pictures of your body. A contrast dye is sometimes injected to help blood vessels show up.

DCIS (DUCTAL CARCINOMA IN SITU): A precancerous step before breast cancer, commonly found around or within your breast cancer.

DEEP INFERIOR EPIGASTRIC PERFORATOR (DIEP) FLAP: A type of "free" tissue reconstruction that is not joined to the original donor site with a pedicle or fixed blood supply.

DELAYED RECONSTRUCTION: A surgical procedure performed to recreate a breast, done some time after the mastectomy treatment for breast cancer.

DONOR SITE: The part of the body from where healthy tissue is moved to another part of the body (usually the chest wall) after a mastectomy.

DOSIMETRIST: A specially trained radiation therapist who calculates the angles and doses of the treatment prescribed by your radiation oncologist.

DUCTAL CARCINOMA IN SITU: see "DCIS"

DUCTS: Tube-like passage that bring breast milk from the lobules to the nipple.

ENDOMETRIAL CANCER: Cancer of the womb.

ESTROGEN: A female hormone that is used in the brain and in female parts of the body such as the breast, womb, and vagina.

ESTROGEN RECEPTOR: A type of antenna inside the nerve centre or "nucleus" of a breast cancer cell or normal cell that binds to estrogen in the bloodstream and allows it to work inside the cell.

ESTROGEN RECEPTOR (ER)-POSITIVE: Hormone sensitive cancer cells that contain the estrogen receptor.

EXTENSIVE INTRADUCTAL COMPONENT (EIC): A type of breast cancer that is surrounded by a lot of pre-cancer or DCIS.

EXTERNAL-BEAM RADIATION: Usually produced by a linear accelerator to kill cancer cells.

EXTRANODAL SPREAD OR EXTENSION (EXTRACAPSULAR SPREAD): When cancer spreads from the inside of a lymph gland through its surrounding capsule to the adjacent fat in your armpit.

EXTRAVASATION: The spillage of chemotherapy into the skin surrounding a vein, rather than remaining inside the vein. Extravasation can cause tissue damage.

FALSE NEGATIVE: A test result (such as a sentinel node biopsy) that shows no cancer present when in fact you actually have cancer that went detected.

FIBROSIS: Scarring and thickening that can occur after radiation therapy, often around a scar where a boost is given, around the pectoralis major muscle, or around a breast implant (after a mastectomy).

FINE NEEDLE (ASPIRATION) BIOPSY: The sampling of breast tissue with a thin needle to suck out cells for examination by a pathologist using a microscope. It may not be as accurate as a core biopsy but it is quicker to perform and can be done using standard needles used for taking blood.

FLAP RECONSTRUCTION: A breast reconstruction involving normal tissue from another part of the body that remains connected to the blood supply from the original or donor location by a flap or pedicle.

FRACTION: A daily dose of or attendance for radiation.

FREE FLAP: A type of flap reconstruction where the tissue is separated from the original donor site and reconnected to the chest area using microsurgery.

FROZEN SECTION: A quick method for a pathologist to examine possible cancerous tissue while you're asleep during an operation. This is often done on a sentinel node, but it's not routinely used except when a mastectomy is planned and a diagnosis has not been firmly established before your surgery.

GLANDS: A term for lymph nodes surrounding your breast in the axilla, internal mammary chain or supra-clavicular fossa. (see "IMC" and "SCF")

GLUTEAL FLAP: A type of breast reconstruction that uses part of your buttock.

GOOGLE SCHOLAR: Part of the Google suite of products that allows users to search for academic works.

GOSERELIN: A manufactured version of luteinizing hormone releasing hormone, or LHRH, branded as Zoladex. It slows the production of estrogen to a level seen during menopause. Goserelin's side effects are similar to the symptoms of menopause.

GRADE: A measure of how slow (low grade) or fast (high grade) a cancer is growing. A grade 1 tumor is slower growing and looks more ordered under a microscope than a grade 3 tumor.

GRAY: A dose unit of radiation therapy. One Gray = 100 rads. (see "RAD")

HEMATOMA: A lump caused by a collection of blood beneath the skin, usually with a surrounding bruise.

HER2 RECEPTOR: A receptor on the surface of all cells known as a human epidermal growth factor receptor 2, which regulates the growth of cells. HER2 positivity or over-expression refers to having an excessive number of HER2 receptors on your breast cancer cells. This occurs in about one in five women with breast cancer, and these tumors tend to grow quicker than HER2-negative tumors.

HERCEPTIN (TRASTUZUMAB): A drug used to bind to the HER2 receptor to prevent it from binding to circulating growth factors in the blood that can cause excessive cell growth.

HISTOLOGIC GRADE: see "GRADE"

HORMONE POSITIVE: see "estrogen receptor (ER)-positive"

HORMONE REPLACEMENT THERAPY (HRT): Tablets taken to replace a woman's natural hormones after menopause. More recently has been called "hormone therapy" or "HT".

HYPERPLASIA: A change in the lining of the ducts in your breast where they increase in number and start to heap up on each other.

IMC: see "INTERNAL MAMMARY CHAIN"

IMMUNO-HISTOCHEMISTRY (or IHC) stain: A chemical stain used by a pathologist to work out whether a specific cell or receptor (such as HER2 or ER) is present in the tissue.

IMMEDIATE RECONSTRUCTION: A surgical procedure or procedures performed to recreate a breast, done at the same time as a mastectomy.

IMPLANT: "see BREAST PROSTHESIS"

IN-SITU HYBRIDIZATION (ISH) TEST: A more accurate test than the IHC test used to detect HER2. It takes one to two weeks to complete.

INFILTRATING DUCTAL CARCINOMA: The most common type of invasive breast cancer, wherein the cells have invaded or infiltrated through the breast duct wall.

INFRA-CLAVICULAR GLANDS: Glands or nodes located under the clavicle or breastbone.

INTERNAL MAMMARY CHAIN (IMC): The lymph glands behind the breastbone or sternum where breast cancer can spread.

INVASIVE CARCINOMA: Cancer cells that have invaded through the duct or lobule of the breast.

INVASIVE LOBULAR CARCINOMA: The second most common type of breast cancer, which starts in the lobules of the breast where milk is normally made after pregnancy.

IN VITRO FERTILIZATION (IVF): The production of a "test tube baby" by collecting an egg, fertilizing it in a test tube with sperm from your partner or a donor, and then freezing it for later use.

ISOLATED TUMOR CELLS (ITCs): Single cells or small clusters of cells not greater than 0.2 mm in largest dimension and classified as pN0(i) in an axillary sentinel node. These are usually not seen by the naked eye but picked up using specials stains or chemicals called immuno-histochemistry (or IHC) stain.

LANGER'S LINES: The natural lines or creases all over the skin. Surgical wounds made parallel to Langer's lines generally heal better and produce less scarring than those that are perpendicular or cut across Langer's lines.

LAPATINIB (TYKERB): A pill taken once daily for HER2-positive breast cancer that has come back; usually combined with chemotherapy.

LATISSIMUS DORSI MUSCLE FLAP: A tissue reconstruction using part of the muscle around your shoulder.

LINEAR ACCELERATOR: A machine that produces high-energy X-rays to destroy cancer cells. It can produce penetrating X-rays or less-penetrating electrons.

LOBULES: The "leaves" connected to the top of the breast ducts that expand and produce milk after pregnancy.

LOCAL RECURRENCE: cancer coming back in the breast after breast conservation, or on the chest wall or surrounding lymph glands after a mastectomy

LUMPECTOMY: Surgical removal of a breast cancer with a healthy margin of normal breast; is usually followed by radiation to the remaining portion of the breast.

LYMPH: Fluid composed of white cells, blood products, and digested food, which helps to fight infection. Lymph is carried throughout the body by the lymphatic system to the lymph glands.

LYMPH GLANDS: Tissues in the lymphatic system that act as filters to fight infection or cancer. These may be felt under the arm if you have breast cancer.

LYMPH NODES: see "LYMPH GLANDS"

LYMPH VESSELS: see "lymphatic system"

LYMPHATIC VESSEL INVASION: SEE "LYMPHOVASCULAR INVASION"

LYMPHATIC SYSTEM: Small vessels, called lymphatics, that carry lymph fluid all around the body, including the breast.

LYMPHATICS: see "LYMPHATIC SYSTEM"

LYMPHEDEMA: Swelling of the arm after treatment to the armpit because of blocked lymphatics causing a backup of fluid.

LYMPHOSCINTIGRAPHY (LYMPHATIC MAPPING): The use of radioactive dye that is taken up by lymphatics and visible on a special camera called a gamma camera. This is done the night before or on the same day as a sentinel node biopsy.

LYMPHOVASCULAR INVASION (LVI): A term used by pathologists to describe the presence of cancer cells in the lymphatics around your breast cancer.

MACRO-METASTASIS: Cancer that is easily visible without special IHC stains in a lymph node or gland.

MACROSCOPIC REPORT: The part of your pathology report that describes what is seen by the pathologist with the naked eye before he or she cuts up the specimen and looks at your cancer with a microscope.

MAMMOGRAM: A breast X-ray routinely done in two directions to characterize a lump, or as a screening test for breast cancer.

MARGIN: The edge of the tissue removed during a lumpectomy. A positive margin has invasive cancer cells or DCIS extending to the edge.

MASTECTOMY: The surgical removal of your entire breast.

MEDICAL ONCOLOGIST: A doctor who specializes in treating cancer with chemotherapy drugs or hormone drugs.

MEDLINE: An electronic index of citations in medical journals from 1950 to the present, with a focus on the biomedical sciences.

MEDULLARY CARCINOMA: A special type of infiltrating breast cancer that is noted by its well-defined edge between the tumor and the surrounding normal tissue. It tends to have a good prognosis.

META-ANALYSIS A statistical methods where the results of many smaller studies are lumped together to determine whether a specific treatment is beneficial or not.

METASTATIC DISEASE Cancer that has spread beyond the breast and lymph glands to another part of the body.

MICRO-METASTASES: Tumor deposits greater than 0.2 mm but not greater than 2.0 mm in dimension in the lymph glands.

MICROSCOPIC REPORT: The part of your pathology report that describes what is seen by the pathologist when sections of your tumor are examined after magnification with a microscope.

MITOSIS: The process of cell division wherein one cells divides into two.

MITOTIC RATE: A measure taken into account when a tumor is graded, wherein the pathologists counts how many cells dividing into two he or she can see in your tumor.

MONOCLONAL ANTIBODY: Manmade antibodies that are designed to lock onto or target certain receptors such as HER2. to deliver treatments directly to the cancer, rather than use chemotherapy treatments that attack normal cells as well.

MUCINOUS CARCINOMA: An uncommon type of breast cancer also known as colloid carcinoma because the cancer cells produce mucus.

MULTICENTRIC CANCER: The presence of two or more cancers in different quadrants of the breast.

MULTIDISCIPLINARY TEAM: A team of doctors and other health care professionals who work and communicate with each other about the best possible treatment for your individual situation.

MULTIFOCAL CANCER: The presence of two or more cancers in the same quadrant of the breast.

NEO-ADJUVANT: Adjuvant therapy given before surgery, such as chemotherapy or hormonal treatment.

NEUTROPENIA: A disorder of the blood, with low levels of the most common and important white cell called the neutrophil.

NODES: SEE "LYMPH GLANDS"

NUCLEAR GRADE: This is how abnormal the nucleus (or control center) of the cancer cell looks. This is scored in a range from 1 to 3.

OCCULT BREAST CANCER: Breast cancer presenting as a lump under the armpit without evidence of the cancer in the breast.

OOPHORECTOMY: Removal of both ovaries and usually the fallopian tubes that connect the ovaries to the uterus or womb.

OSTEOPENIA: Weakening of the bones that occurs as you get older or from lack of estrogen due to menopause or drugs such as aromatase inhibitors; less severe than osteoporosis.

OSTEOPOROSIS: Weakening of the bones that occurs as you get older or from lack of estrogen due to menopause or drugs such as aromatase inhibitors.

PLASTIC SURGEON: A surgeon who specializes in breast reconstructive procedures.

PORT: An access site connected to a large vein in the body and used to give chemotherapy instead of inserting multiple needles into the veins of your arm.

POST-MASTECTOMY RADIATION THERAPY: The use of radiation to the chest wall and/or glands after a mastectomy.

PROGESTERONE RECEPTOR (PR): A hormone receptor on the cell that binds the hormone progesterone. Tumors with plenty of PR are more responsive to hormonal treatment than those without.

PROGNOSIS: An estimation of the potential survival rate at a given point of time with or without treatment.

PUBMED: A website for finding academic publications of your treating doctor.

RADIATION DOSE: SEE "GRAY"

RADIATION ONCOLOGIST: A doctor who specializes in treating cancer with radiation therapy. Also known as a radiotherapist.

RADIATION THERAPIST: A specially trained person who works the equipment that delivers radiation therapy.

RADIATION THERAPY (RADIOTHERAPY): The treatment of disease by radiation.

RADS: The metric unit for a Gray.

REDUCTION MAMMOPLASTY: A plastic surgical procedure that reduces the size of your normal breast by removing skin, fat, and breast tissue. Always make sure that your surgeon sends the normal tissue for pathology testing.

SARCOMA: A type of cancer that forms from the surrounding or connective tissue such as muscle, fat, bone, cartilage, or blood vessels. A sarcoma occurs very rarely after treatment of breast cancer in a swollen arm or a breast previously treated with radiation.

SCF: SEE "SUPRA-CLAVICULAR FOSSA (SCF)"

SELECTIVE ESTROGEN RECEPTOR MODULATOR (SERM): A drug that acts like estrogen on some tissues but blocks the effect of estrogen on others. Tamoxifen (Nolvadex) and raloxifene (Evista) are two examples of SERMs.

SENTINEL NODES: A type of "guardian" lymph gland through which the lymphatic vessels drain first before connecting to other lymph glands. There are usually one to three sentinel nodes that drain each breast.

SENTINEL NODE BIOPSY: Removal of the sentinel node on the same side of the breast cancer after "sentinel node mapping", and if that is clear, no further lymph glands are taken.

SENTINEL NODE MAPPING: Identification of the sentinel lymph node(s), by injection of a radioactive substance, blue dye, or both near the tumor. A scanner called a gamma camera is used to find the sentinel lymph node(s) before surgery with an X-ray. During surgery, the surgeon uses a probe to find the lymph node(s) containing the radioactive substance or looks for nodes which have stained blue. The surgeon then removes the sentinel node(s) to check for the presence of cancer either quickly while you are anesthetized ("quick-test") or thoroughly in the week after your surgery.

SEROMA: A short-lived fluid collection that occurs after surgery in your breast, chest wall, or armpit.

SEROUS FLUID: Straw-colored fluid that leaks from lymphatics and small blood vessels following surgery into tissues.

SIMPLE MASTECTOMY: SEE "TOTAL MASTECTOMY"

SIMULATION: A session where your radiation treatment setup is mocked up for your shape and size, and then a CT scan is done to map out your internal organs.

SKIN-SPARING MASTECTOMY: Mastectomy performed by removing the breast tissue through a small scar without removing all of the overlying skin. The natural shape and contour of the breast is recreated using either an implant or tissue flap.

STAGE 1, 2, 3, 4: The degree of spread of all cancers is usually classified by four stages of increasing severity. For patients with breast cancer, stage 1 means that it is localized to the breast and stage 4 means that it has spread to other areas of the body.

STERNUM: The breastbone.

SUB-CUTICULAR STITCHES: Dissolving sutures that are used to bring the skin together after surgery and are buried under the skin. They look and scar better than a "railroad track" type of stitch, which is external, needs removal, and leaves a more obvious scar.

SUPERFICIAL INFERIOR EPIGASTRIC ARTERY (SIEA) FLAP: A type of "free" tissue reconstruction wherein the tissue is not joined to the original donor site with a pedicle or fixed blood supply.

SUPRA-CLAVICULAR FOSSA (SCF): Lymph glands that are found just above the breastbone (clavicle).

SUPRA-STERNAL NOTCH: The curved notch formed by the top end of your breastbone (sternum) and the ends of the breastbone (clavicle); always used as a reference point to mark the center of your body lengthwise when planning or treating with radiation.

SURGEON: A doctor who specializes in removing cancer with surgery. Some surgeons are called surgical oncologists if they specialize in surgery for many cancers, or breast surgeons if they specifically specialize in breast cancer. Some surgeons are general surgeons, who may have an interest in breast cancer but may not necessarily work in a multidisciplinary team.

TAMOXIFEN: A drug that binds to estrogen receptors on cells to stop them from binding with circulating estrogen. Estrogen can make some breast cancer cells grow, and tamoxifen can starve these cells of estrogen and help them shrink or die.

TELANGIECTASIA: Prominent blood vessels that may appear in areas of skin that received a higher dose of radiation, such as over your scar or under your breast.

TERMINAL DUCT LOBULAR UNIT: The part of the breast duct that joins the lobule, which is thought to be where breast cancer usually begins.

THROMBOCYTOPENIA: The presence of low numbers of platelets in the blood, which can cause bruising.

THRUSH: A fungal infection, usually of the tongue and inside your cheeks, identified by white plaque that can occur when your immunity is depressed during chemotherapy or sometimes as a side effect of antibiotics. Thrush can also occur elsewhere, including the vagina.

TISSUE EXPANDER: A breast implant inserted under the skin and muscles of the chest which is expanded over a few weeks by repeated injections of salt water to form a mound shaped like a breast after a mastectomy.

TOTAL MASTECTOMY: Removal of the entire breast without the underlying muscle or the lymph glands (lymph nodes) in the armpit (axilla).

TRANSVERSE RECTUS ABDOMINUS MUSCLE (TRAM) FLAP: A type of "pedicle" tissue reconstruction wherein the donor tissue is joined to the blood supply of the original donor site in the tummy area. By using tissue from your tummy, a "tummy tuck" is a bonus. Because it is fat and muscle, it feels more natural than an internal prosthesis or implant.

TRIPLE-NEGATIVE BREAST CANCER: A type of invasive carcinoma, associated with a poorer prognosis, that is HER2-negative, ER-negative, and PR-negative.

TUBULAR CARCINOMA: A rare type of invasive carcinoma associated with a good prognosis.

TUBULE FORMATION: One of the components (with mitotic rate and nuclear grade) for determining a cancer's overall grade. With higher-grade cancers, there are only a few or no tubules.

TUMOR BED: The area left behind after a cancer is removed; it is often is at risk for cancer cells being left behind and therefore needs a higher dose of radiation, or a boost.

TYROSINE KINASE INHIBITORS (TKIs): A monoclonal antibody, such as lapatinib, that also targets the HER2 receptor.

ULTRASOUND: High frequency sound waves used to locate a tumor inside the body. A picture is shown on a computer or video screen and shows if a tumor is solid or contains fluid (a cyst).

ZOLADEX: see "goserelin"

Index

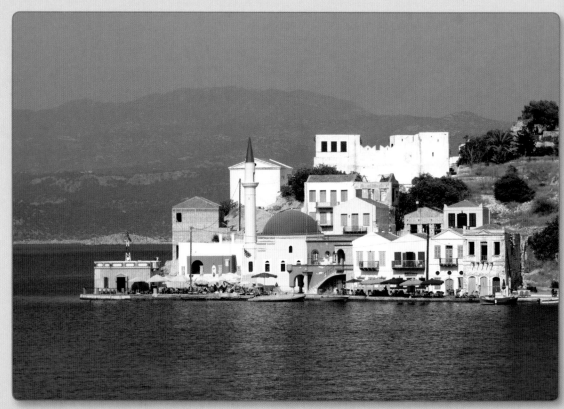

My Thoughts and Notes

Write down your thoughts, feelings, or questions here, in the margins of the book or consider getting a journal or start a blog. Sometimes writing down your worries helps you to work through them. Don't forget to have a glass of champagne or your favorite drink when you have finished your treatment. Stand tall and move forward.

My Thoughts and Notes

My Contacts

Name

Address

Phone No.

Email

My Surgeon

Name

Address

Phone No.

My Radiation Oncologist

Name

Address

Phone No.

My Medical Oncologist

Name

Address

Phone No.

My Breast Care Nurse

Name

Address

Phone No.

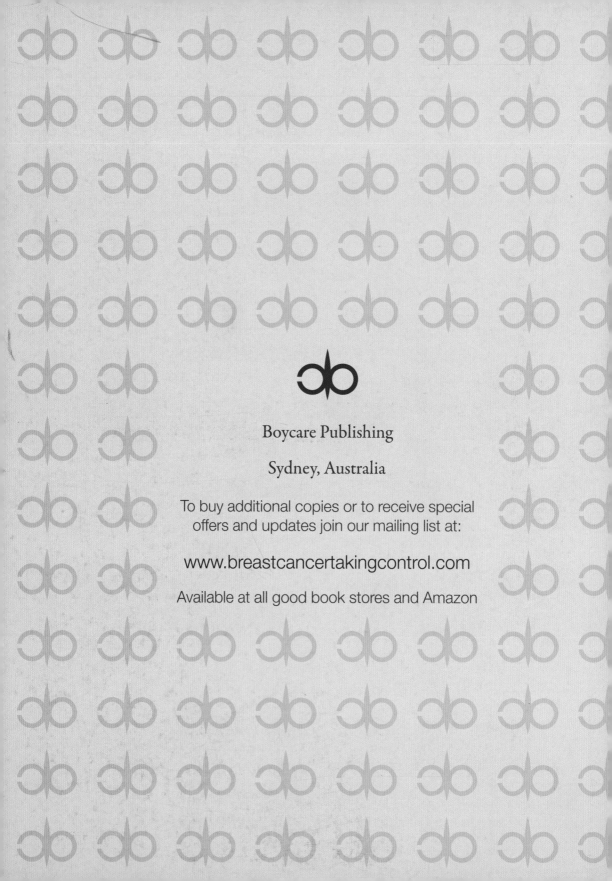

Boycare Publishing

Sydney, Australia

To buy additional copies or to receive special
offers and updates join our mailing list at:

www.breastcancertakingcontrol.com

Available at all good book stores and Amazon